Praise for Lou Paget's Mind-Blowing Techniques

THE LADIES SAY . . .

"My response to my boyfriend's reaction when I first tried these techniques was, 'He must be faking this, it can't feel that good,' but it did! Thank you for this and all the rest we've yet to try."

Mortgage broker, 28, Glendale, California.

"I want you to know that you saved my sister's marriage. She was frustrated after seven years and fearing that the only way to spice things up was to have an affair. You showed her ways to have that kind of excitement in her marriage."

Physician, 37, Chicago, Illinois.

"I couldn't believe that the kind of information that I had looked for for years was actually available—those really nitty-gritty details and tips that others say worked for them. And it's presented so tastefully!!"

Sales executive, 33, Omaha, Nebraska.

"I told my friends, 'You've *got* to hear this woman. Her techniques will give you power where you didn't know you had it. It's a crash course on female sexuality presented with the attitude of Estes' *Women Who Run with the Wolves* delivered by a female John Gray.'"*

Advertising executive, 29, Buffalo, New York.

*author of Men Are from Mars, Women Are from Venus

"My husband's plans for a solo European business trip changed the night after your seminar. He said, 'You're coming, I can't leave you behind.' You've changed my life—and my husband's."

Movie producer, 38, Beverly Hills, California.

"I now have the freedom to believe that if it feels good, it *is* good. There is a belief in *myself* that has started to emerge, rather than a belief in the ideas that I grew up with."

Computer programming vice president, 36, Sacramento, California.

"I now feel like I have this terrific secret. Like I own something very special and new, and should I choose to do so, I can bestow it on any lucky recipient. It has given me a confidence best described as 'I'm so hot, and you don't even know it.'"

Divorced single mother, 44, Beverly Hills, California.

"I waited a week before I did anything with what I'd learned. When I told my boyfriend 'I think you're ready,' it was about me being ready, not him. That week of waiting was like a week of foreplay . . . and we had *sooo* much fun. He now tells everyone I am the sexiest woman he knows. And now we can talk in ways we couldn't before."

Chief financial officer, 37, Seattle, Washington.

"The next night I tried it out on my new boyfriend and he said it was kind of frightening how good I was. He said I paid attention to all the right places, but that it was mostly the enthusiasm and intensity that made it so great."

Editor, 22, Los Angeles, California.

THEIR PARTNERS SAY . . .

"There is nothing to compare her to, no one even comes close. Spoiled isn't the term I'd use—ruined is more like it."

Novelist, 29, Boston, Massachusetts.

"I've been with many women and I thought I'd seen it all. No one even approaches her hand jobs. My girlfriend now does me better than I do myself."

Executive film producer, 48, Los Angeles, California.

"This was the best four-hour investment my wife ever made for our relationship."

Financial analyst, 35, New York, New York.

"At first I couldn't believe that she went to this and afterwards I thanked God."

Studio executive, 28, Los Angeles, California.

"I cannot thank you enough for what you gave my fiancée. We were already really open about sex but this took us to another level. And we were amazed at what we thought we knew and didn't."

Printer, 44, Indianapolis, Indiana.

How to Be a
Great Lover

How to Be a
Great Lover

GIRLFRIEND-TO-GIRLFRIEND
TOTALLY EXPLICIT
TECHNIQUES THAT WILL
BLOW HIS MIND

Lou Paget

Broadway Books / New York

Broadway Books titles may be purchased for business or promotional use or for special sales. For information, please write to: Special Markets Department, Random House, Inc., 1540 Broadway, New York, NY 10036.

BROADWAY BOOKS and its logo, a letter B bisected on the diagonal, are trademarks of Broadway Books, a division of Random House, Inc.

Library of Congress Cataloging-in-Publication Data
Paget, Lou.
How to be a great lover: girlfriend-to-girlfriend totally explicit techniques that will blow his mind / by Lou Paget.
p.   cm.
ISBN 0-7679-0287-4 (hc)
1. Sexual excitement—Popular works.   2. Women—Sexual behavior—Popular works.   3. Sex—Popular works.   I. Title.
HQ21 P14   1999
306.7—dc21   98-41537
                                                      CIP

FIRST EDITION

Designed by Jennifer Ann Daddio

99 00 01 02 03 10 9 8 7 6 5 4 3 2 1

TO BRYAN THALHEIMER

You shared the magic of your attitude and information.

And without whom this would not have been possible.

TO ALL OF THE LADIES IN THE SEMINARS

This book is a dedication to your sharing.

When you give from your heart you give of the gold.

You can't be thanked enough.

Acknowledgments

I asked a many-times-published friend, "What is the best thing about writing a book?" He responded, "Doing the acknowledgments and dedication pages." You know what? He was right.

THE SUPPORT TEAM

To Dede, Lisa, and Michelle, without whom I couldn't have stayed the course.

To Sherry, Katerena, Carolynn, Tammy, and Buffy—the other ladies in my family, for their unending, uncomplicated, and sweet, sweet support.

Jessica Kalkin, Matthew Davidge, Ariel Sotolongo my "HCB", Maura McAniff, Rebecca Clemons, Priscilla Wallace, Sandra Beck, Gail Harrington, Raymond Davi, Jay Rosen, Alan Cochran, Michael Levin, Peter Greenberg, Kendra King, Joyce Lyons, Nance Mitchell, Stacy Rozsa, Peter Redgrove, Elizabeth Hall, Morley Winnick, Marianne Huning, Bob Linn, T. J. Rozsa, Greg Pryor, Marsha and Wayne Williams, Mark Helm, and all at Women's Referral Service (WRS).

THE CREATIVE TEAM

Joan S., who gave me the idea and insisted I do it.

Catherine McEvily Harris and Billie Fitzpatrick, who took my voice and masterfully turned it into words.

Debra Goldstein: an agent like you is every author's dream.

Lauren Marino: THE editor. The Buddha-like calm in the middle of the storm. She has one of the best laughs.

Ann Campbell, assistant editor, and Nancy Peske, copy editor.

All at Broadway Books and Creative Culture.

THE RESEARCH & DEVELOPMENT TEAM

Penelope Hitchcock, DVM, Jacqueline Snow, MN, CNP, Eric Daar, MD, Bernie Zilbergeld, PhD, Bryce Britton, MS, Ron McAllister, PhD, Nancy Breuer, Lynne Gabriel, Uri Peles, MD, Dennis Paradise, Norm Zafman, Shannon Foley.

Contents

How to Be a
Great Lover

Chapter One

The Kama Lou Tra

HOW I CAME TO TEACH
THE SEXUALITY SEMINARS

*"I can now throw out the message 'If you're too
experienced or know too much—you're a slut.' I now see
that couldn't be further from the truth. There is such
power in owning one's sexuality and self."*

FEMALE SEMINAR ATTENDEE,

WRITER/PRODUCER, AGE 39

Gathered in a boardroom in an elegant midtown private club,
ten to fifteen women, ranging in age from early twenties to mid-
fifties, stare at the table center. The table itself is laid with sil-
ver flatware, linen napkins, and fresh flowers. It's evening and
the lighting is dim, provoking an air of expectancy.

"Okay ladies, this will be the first of many choices you will
have to make this evening." I stand at the head of a long, rec-
tangular mahogany table.

Some of the women are dressed in couture suits; others are
dressed more casually, in slacks; others are still more casual,
decked in a downtown hip look. The women are staring rather

mutely at the center of the table, in which are placed a selection of what I affectionately call "instructional products" (better known as dildos).

"Without being overly PC, please select the color of your choice—white, black, or mulatto—and the size you prefer—8-inch, 7-inch, 6-inch, or the ever-so-popular 5-inch executive model."

I hear a few peals of laughter and then I smile at the newcomers and say again, "Ladies, go ahead and choose an instructional product."

A tall, lanky woman in her mid-forties says, "Do I have to choose what I have at home?"

Gales of laughter follow. The women look around at each other and can't believe they are laughing so hard. I know now, after almost six years of conducting The Sexuality Seminars across the U.S. and in Canada, that this is the ice-breaking moment, when the women who have come to learn more about sex, and specifically, to learn how to become a better lover, begin to relax.

How to Be a Great Lover is a cumulative extension of these seminars and includes not only what I have learned from my research, but also what I have learned from the many women who have attended the seminars. Throughout the book, you will hear their voices, as well as the voices of their men, sharing their experiences—woman to woman. As one woman, a fifty-five-year-old housewife from Seattle, told me, "I found out learning about sex isn't just for my children's generation. After my husband's death, I am dating again and at my age, I HAVE to know about safe sex."

I want to be absolutely clear about the *spirit* with which this book was written. It was never my intent to sit down and create a book about how to please a man. While there is no point in arguing the fact that the man in your life will be a major beneficiary of the information found here, the real purpose is threefold: to empower you as a woman, heighten the intimacy of your romantic relationship, and enable you and your partner to enjoy yourselves in intense new ways.

While biology may have graced us with a basic understanding of how to have sex, we are not necessarily born great lovers. We learn to be great lovers. And I have always believed that anything worth doing is worth doing well. Wouldn't you agree that the better we are at something, the more we enjoy doing it? Sex is no different. It shouldn't be an experience just to get *through*, but rather an experience to be relished from beginning to end. For that to happen, you've got to know what you're doing.

I also believe that every woman has the right to be sexually proficient. You'll find that knowing what to do to your man's body can provide you with as much power as it does pleasure. And contrary to what we've been made to feel in the past, there never has, nor ever *will* be anything unladylike about being masterful in the bedroom. The truth is, being sexually savvy is no less a part of being a woman than motherhood, and learning how to be a great lover is about excelling in all areas of womanhood.

It's for these reasons, as well as the demand from the women in the seminars, that I decided to write a book that teaches women the art of sex, and I hope to give you extraordinary tools that will enable you to please your lover beyond his wildest expectations.

The first place most of us learned about sex was in the company of our girlfriends. It is certainly the first place we *laughed* about it. Most of us can vividly recall squirming in uncomfortable silence while our mothers struggled to tell us the facts of life, or how we sunk deep into our chairs during health class, praying the teacher would spare us the humiliation of having to discuss the subject out loud. At the same time, we can also remember those wonderful Friday nights, sitting pajama-clad in a circle of five or six of our closest pals, listening intently as the girls with the older sisters shared amazing stories about what they'd seen and overheard through keyholes. We absorbed their tales as if they were gospel, giving far more credence to their words than those of our mothers and teachers. We may have giggled and acted shocked, but secretly we couldn't wait to experience sex for ourselves. Indeed, sex seemed like a fabulous, exciting adventure.

Years later, when we were finally ready to act on our exciting adventure, we knew little more about how to proceed than what we could remember from the long, lost tales of those older sisters. We may have grown more comfortable with the thought of *having* sex, but we weren't any closer to really knowing what to do. Complicating matters further was the feeling that there was no place we could go for information about *how* to learn to do it, much less how to be *good* at it. Neither our mothers nor our health teachers ever included any specific how-tos in their sex education chats. We can't blame our mothers; I'd bet that if they *weren't* ignorant about techniques, they would still be *way* too embarrassed to get into the specifics with their daughters. And I doubt a teacher who taught sexual technique would last long in any school district.

As confusing and difficult as it was for us to discuss sex back when we were young women, it only got worse as we got older. Not knowing what to do sexually as a young woman is uncomfortable and at times embarrassing, but it doesn't compare to the inadequacy we feel in having to ask questions on the subject once we've passed the age when were already *supposed* to know.

Like me, many women have always felt embarrassed, even ashamed, for desiring to know more about sex or to improve their skills in this area. After all, what kind of young lady would want to be good in bed? In other words, how does she *admit* she wants to be good in bed, and remain a lady? For me, this dilemma goes back to the way I was raised: don't talk about sex, don't think about it, and above all, don't do it. So with that as my psychological imprimatur, how was I going to learn about sex? Men could learn how to be great lovers through experience. In fact, they were given kudos for it. What *women* were given for experience in this area, however, was a reputation. There's a complicated double bind here: on one end of the sexuality continuum, under what I call the "Don't Umbrella," we have the "don't ask because it's bad" attitude. On the other end of the continuum, we are taught that sex is a form of manipulation we should use to control our man.

Neither of these options ever made sense to me. I wanted something in the middle: practical, real information that would enable me to feel comfortable sexually. I believe that sex should be an expression and celebration of my feelings, and all *I* wanted was to be brilliant at sex with the one man of my choice. It didn't seem like too much to ask.

Where do we women *usually* go to develop sexual savviness? As one woman, an accountant from Chicago, said, "For most of us, the level of our sexual prowess is only as good as that of our best lover—and we might have left him behind in high school."

So how do nice girls like us go about learning about sex? The most obvious place is from the man or men in your life, especially those who introduce us to our first sexual experiences. Often men are sexually active at a younger age than women, so we depend on them to show us the ropes. Unfortunately, they usually don't have teaching on their minds. Being goal-oriented, they just want to have an orgasm. If an orgasm is out of the question, their next focus is getting as close to it as possible. Young men like to see how far we'll allow them to go. They may know how to do it, but not necessarily how to do it *well*. So ideally, it is in a long-term relationship, where we (finally) may feel comfortable enough to ask questions and experiment, that we learn the most.

Another route to sexual knowledge is to practice on as many different men's bodies as possible, and perhaps, through trial and error, we may arrive at some confidence in our know-how. However, I believe that, with what we know today about sexually transmitted diseases, that is not a wise choice. The risk of AIDS and other STDs lurk dangerously close to home. But, if you're like most of us, becoming intimate with lots of different men is something you just may not be comfortable with, and for those of us in a committed relationship, this isn't an option at all.

For me, once I decided I wanted to learn more about what to do sexually, I went searching for a source that would help me master these skills, just as I had mastered other skills in my life. As I mentioned before, I'm a firm believer in the adage that *anything* you're going to be doing regularly is worth doing well. And of all the things a woman should want to be her best at, loving a man intimately seemed a logical priority. At the time, I was on the brink of my first truly romantic adult relationship with a man I'd hoped to be with forever (it didn't turn out that way, but that's another story altogether). And with my unwavering curiosity, I began a determined quest for reliable information about sex that made sense to me and wouldn't infringe on my values. The first place I turned was to books, and by virtue of its erotic reputation, my first stop was *The Kama Sutra*.

Long considered one of the oldest and most definitive written sources on sexual technique and pleasure, *The Kama Sutra* was originally compiled in the fourth century A.D. It was put together by a Brahmin and religious scholar named Vatsyayana, who gathered his material from texts dating back to the fourth century B.C. Since then, the work has been updated and appended several times and translated into many different languages. I'd heard about *The Kama Sutra* for years, and it always evoked a vision of sensual eroticism in my mind. When I finally opened the book and began to read, I was very surprised, for two reasons. The first factor that shocked me about this engaging and abundant work was the uninhibited view of sexuality in ancient India. The book's depiction of sexual acts between men and women made me wonder why and how sex ever got to be the taboo subject it has become in modern times. Furthermore, *The Kama Sutra* openly and unabashedly covers such topics as romance, marriage, adultery, bigamy, group sex, prostitution, sadomasochism, male and female homosexuality, and transvestism.

The second aspect of *The Kama Sutra* that struck me is the uselessness of its information for contemporary women. This is not to say the book isn't fascinating, because it is. It's also highly entertaining. Furthermore, *The Kama Sutra* is a beautifully detailed representation of this antediluvian Indian culture. But rather than serving as a guide to sexual technique for both sexes as it has been billed, it's more accurately a coming-of-age handbook for upper-class adolescent boys and young men in fourth-century India. *The Kama Sutra* discusses what were then the three aims in a man's life (virtue, wealth, love) and how they can be acquired through the mastery of erotic touch. For example, the book describes the conduct of a well-bred townsman (he must bathe regularly and keep a *separate* bed in his room to use with prostitutes), as well as explains the fine art of seducing a girl (including how to scratch, bite, and administer blows to her back and head). The book even provides advice and proper etiquette for those particularly delicate situations such as dealing with more than one wife at a time, and seducing *other* men's wives.

The Indian culture depicted in *The Kama Sutra* clearly placed great value on sexual expression and fulfillment. Erotic pleasure was considered divine, and the desire to provide it was every bit as consuming as the desire to receive it. Still, *The Kama Sutra* has a decidedly male perspective. While much attention is given to the techniques of pleasuring a woman, it is obvious the information recorded here was gained through observation rather than conversation. It is unlikely that the women on whom these writings are based were actually consulted about what it is that puts them into a divine state. Let me give you an example. Part Two of *The Kama Sutra* is devoted to "amorous advances." The following is excerpted from the chapter on embraces:

> *Lying on his side, either he rests his best limb on her as on a brood mare, or else lying on top of her, the part of his body below the navel resting on the girl's pubis, he presses his instrument against her without penetrating her. At that moment, the girl's sex opens out, overexcited, particularly if she has a large organ. Thrusting his groin firmly against the girl's pubis, he seizes her by the hair and stays crouched over her in order to scratch, bite, and strike her.*

Does that sound like something pleasurable to you? Even those who enjoy sex a little bit rough at times, or who view spanking as something erotic, wouldn't take kindly to being pinned down like a brood mare in order to be scratched, bitten, and hit. Still, I don't think that women at the time, unlike in modern India, were as disrespected as they were misunderstood. In spite of such slights toward women, in Vatsyayana's original version of *The Kama Sutra,* women were nonetheless held in high esteem. The book makes it very clear that, from a man's perspective, being desired by a woman was considered an honor, and the seduction of a woman was a form of art. However, art, as we all well know, is and always has been a very subjective phenomenon. As the saying goes, *One man's trash is another man's treasure*. Or, as the case may be, one man's perspective isn't necessarily another woman's pleasure.

My reason for sharing this particular excerpt from *The Kama Sutra* was to show you how easy it is to get irrelevant information in the area of sexual technique. And while I learned a lot about fourth-century Indian culture and picked up some very vivid tips on positions from it, *The Kama Sutra* was neither what I expected, nor what I needed. And so my quest for practical sexual knowledge continued.

Secret from Lou's Archives

Ways women can gauge certain male features: 1) the length from the tip of his index finger to the base of the palm of his hand indicates erect penis size; 2) the longer or wider the moon on his thumbnail, the longer or wider his penis will be. As one seminar attendee said, "It makes the ride on the subway so much more interesting!"

I soon found other books, some of which provided a modicum of useful information. I was in search of information about what men found most exciting and why, and perhaps even more importantly, what techniques were known to be successful, in easy-to-understand explanations, telling me exactly how sexual acts were done. Where did people put their thumbs? What did they do with their tongues? What were they actually doing? In bookstores and libraries, mostly what I saw were tomes on sexual history with pictures or drawings of men and women in positions that seemed unnatural, uncomfortable, and in no way right for me. Even if I could have followed the accompanying instructions, I felt certain one or both of us would have ended up in traction much sooner than in sexual bliss.

In all fairness, there were a few bright lights on the horizon. Books such as *The Sensuous Woman* by "J," *The Happy Hooker* by Xaviera Hollander, and Alex Comfort's *The Joy of Sex* presented information in a way that appealed to me—as if sexual interaction and the desire to be good at it was something perfectly natural for everyone. In these books, the bodies depicted seemed like they belonged to normal people, and the sexual scenarios also seemed realistic, like they possibly could have taken place somewhere other than Fantasy Island. And I did learn something: before reading *The Sensuous Woman,* I had never even heard of oral sex!

But as much as I enjoyed all three of these books, reading them was like watching television on mute: the pictures were helpful, but there weren't enough specific details on how to achieve these results in my own bedroom.

The next place I went for practical advice was to the movies. While Hollywood does a good job of providing ideas on how to create a sensual atmosphere in scenes in some of the R-rated movies, when it comes to actual sex scenes, directors cut away to exuberant facial expressions, followed by two people basking in the afterglow, without offering a single lesson in how that radiant afterglow was achieved. When the movies ended, I felt frustrated by the mere thought of the actors having information that I didn't. The fact that the men and women involved were only acting did little to quench my thirst for their knowledge, whether it was real or imaginary.

In my search for sexual know-how, I turned next to pornography. This is a $1-billion-a-year business and the majority of consumers are men. Therefore, porn movies are a logical place to research what turns men on sexually. And I must say, you do get to *see* what's going on in porn films. Unlike in mainstream movies, an X rating pretty much guarantees that all the action takes place *on top of* the sheets, rather than underneath them. But after watching a few of them, I found the films all began to merge and look alike and I was as bored as I was saddened.

I was turned off by the way women were represented in most of the films. It wasn't that what they were *doing* felt wrong to me, for I expected to see explicit sexual acts being done in a variety of positions and to hear language not found in my everyday vocabulary. As far as I'm concerned, at times there is a place for even the raunchiest sex between consenting adults. Rather, I was disappointed in the total lack of romance, love, caring, and respect between the men and women depicted in the films.

The sex in porn movies is all performance with no connection of spirits. The men and women barely have personalities. I was sincerely open to looking at all the ways I could be sexually masterful and alluring, but that didn't mean being reduced to a sexual mechanic. Nor did it include sharing my body or my man with other people. That would defeat the purpose of sexual intimacy entirely.

For me, there are at least two problems with porn movies as an education source: first, the objectification of women completely destroys any sense of the intimacy most of us crave in our sexual encounters; and second, porn movies present only a male view, portraying what visually turns men on. There's a small problem: they forgot to consider consulting 50 percent of the participants—us women.

When I have asked men what they get from watching porn

films, they tell me they use them to "get the juices flowing" or "to get ideas for positions." One seasoned infomercial producer told me, "I use them to compare how I'm doing, and measure my performance." But for us women, using porn as a guide to finding out what we like and are comfortable with is at best, inaccurate and at worst, laughable.

So again, I had struck out in my quest to find a useful and appropriate source for further sexual education. I was caught between a rock and a hard place. I really wanted to be good in bed, but not at the expense of my values. I hadn't found anywhere that, for lack of a better term, nice upstanding women could go to in order to learn how to express their love for a man in a physical manner, or to have their sexual questions answered. It just wasn't done.

Finally, at my wit's end, I decided to go straight to the source: enter my dear friend, Bryan. The truth of the matter was that the forever love I mentioned earlier and I had long since broken up, but I was optimistic that at *some* point in my life, I'd get another crack at love and romance. And I wanted to be ready. I could talk to Bryan about anything, and his being gay meant that the subject wasn't the least bit dangerous for either of us. In other words, there was no chance of his leering at me and saying, "*I'll* show you, baby." He empathized with my problem and wanted to point me in the right direction.

Over several cups of café latte at his house, Bryan asked me what it was that I wanted to know, and why I hadn't asked my boyfriend what *he* wanted in bed. I said to him, "Bryan, how can you ask for what you want to know, when you don't even know what that is?" I told him that I was comfortable with my knowledge about intercourse, but it was the *other* stuff men liked that I wanted more information on. The more information I have, the higher my comfort level, and the higher my comfort level, the more confidence I have. I knew that with more knowledge on oral and manual techniques, I'd be able to express my love more creatively, and in a way that better represented the depth of my feelings.

Bryan didn't laugh or make fun of me. All he said was, "Then you've got to know one thing: for me, the key to great sex is in the foreplay." He explained that when it comes to making love, intercourse is just the tip of the iceberg, and that the foundation of amazing lovemaking lies in foreplay. That's where the great lovers are separated from the mediocre ones. This made sense to me. I knew foreplay was the key to exciting sex for *women*, so why shouldn't that be true for men?

As we sat in his house over lattes, Bryan picked up his spoon and told me to do the same with mine. Pretending it was a penis, he showed me what feels good to men. He explained which areas of the penis are extra sensitive, requiring a gentle touch, as well as those areas where more pressure should be applied for maximum results. He also showed me some creative things to do with my hands, tongue, and throat that would create a variety of sensations in just the right places. Bryan's explanations were clear and logical. The great part was that I soon found they didn't suffer in the translation from spoon to penis.

That first real sexual lesson was back in 1985 and to this day, it was the best latte I *ever* had. There was one particular move Bryan showed me that I can honestly say has *never* failed me. And all the women in my seminars who have tried it on *their* men say exactly the same thing. I call it "Ode to Bryan," in memory of my dear friend Bryan who has since passed away. (You'll find out precisely how the "Ode to Bryan" is done in Chapter 6.)

There is no way I could have imagined what kind of impact

that conversation with Bryan would have on my life. I certainly never dreamed it would turn into a career. But the transformation in my way of being with and relating to men was profound. It provided me with the confidence I needed to explore my own sexuality. For a long time, I kept the information to myself. It wasn't intentional; I guess I just didn't realize or think about how many other women could relate to the same frustrations when it came to sexual know-how.

One night in 1993 while visiting with a couple of girlfriends, I got to talking with them about sex, our love lives, and men in general. Somewhere in the midst of the conversation, one of them mentioned that the sex had not been everything she had hoped it would be between her and her fiancé. The problem, she said, was *hers*. Here she was, about to get married, and she had little confidence in her sexual ability beyond intercourse. She was reluctant to try anything at which she might fail. My other friend empathized, sheepishly admitting that she didn't know exactly what to do, either. They both said lack of knowledge made them feel awkward and inhibited in bed. But what were they going to do? There wasn't a place where women who valued their reputations and self-respect could go to learn sexual techniques.

Yes, there is, I told them, wondering to myself if Bryan was looking down from heaven at that moment. *Right here.* I got out three spoons and began to talk. I showed them everything Bryan had shown me, and added a few moves I'd come up with myself. We laughed until the wee hours of the morning, exchanging ideas and sexual anecdotes about all the wrong information we'd gotten in the past. Nothing could have prepared me for what was to follow. Within a week I got phone calls from both of my friends, saying that the things I showed them that night had actually led to dramatic improvements in their sex lives already! They referred to me as The Kama *Lou* Tra and said I should consider going into the business of teaching nice women about sex.

I became interested in learning about and enjoying good sex, but with HIV and AIDS an unfortunate reality, I also wanted to know how to have sex safely. Soon I was holding informal focus groups and the idea of writing a book on safe sex in the nineties began to emerge. In the focus groups, I asked women what questions they had on the subject of sex. Their responses blew me away: I had not been alone in either my curiosity or my lack of knowledge about sex. And while they, too, were concerned about sexual safety, they were, like me, interested in sexual mastery. They believed that being a great lover was very much a part of being a great woman.

That's how it all started. The evolution into The Sexuality Seminars began slowly, with those friends telling other friends about the information they received. Pretty soon I was giving seminars several nights a week after work. After a while, the phone was ringing off the hook and I was getting so many requests that I ended up quitting my regular job and committing full time to developing and giving the workshops. I have to admit that at first, I wasn't comfortable with this new image of myself. It took some getting used to the fact that I was suddenly an expert on sex. Today, as a sex educator, I give seminars all over the country and throughout Canada. The business has expanded beyond women to include seminars for men, couples, and specialty groups such as bridal showers, bachelor parties, and birthdays.

Every seminar is an exchange of ideas. Much like a snowball rolling down a hill, the seminar information base grows with every good idea I hear. There has yet to be one in which I didn't learn something new, and I don't expect there ever will be. So, although I *lead* those seminars, the information I deliver has come from innumerable sources. I can't emphasize enough how much sharing of information goes on in the seminars, and as you read the book, you will hear, see, and feel how the women exchange their ideas, build their knowledge, and develop their confidence in becoming good, dare I say expert, lovers. You'll also hear directly from men: what they like and what turns them on most. I bet some of their responses will indeed surprise you.

The heart and premise of these very confidential seminars (no disrobing is permitted) was to create a safe, respectful place for women to exchange ideas on sexuality that they knew worked. And when women shared what they knew with others it in turn validated and expanded what they already knew. Chances are you will recognize some of these techniques as your own, or very similar to your own. Outstanding! If you find yourself already familiar with any of these techniques, that's great. Simply move on to the next or compare notes with how yours is done. Though I have led these seminars for over five years, I still hear something new in each and every one of them. How? By always staying open and ready to learn. The women who come to the seminars feel the same way. One woman, a Russian émigré, said, "This is my fourth seminar and I can't believe how much I can still learn. I came again for a refresher." At the beginning of the seminar, the ladies think I am the one who knows; by the end, they feel as if they are the ones who know.

How to Be a Great Lover draws on the thousands of interviews I've conducted and scientific research I've reviewed over the past fifteen years, and is a compilation of what I have learned listening to the myriad women who have attended the seminars. The women come to share, listen, and learn, and it's in this spirit that the book is written. The seminars continue to grow, with women learning about them from word of mouth (so far, I have not done any direct marketing).

Secret from Lou's Archives
As men age, they need more stimulation and foreplay. In a way they become more like women.

Regardless of your present experience or level of inhibition, there is something here for you. The book has a lot of fresh ideas about the sensual basics of romantic ambiance, kissing, intercourse, and safety. But the juice is found in the chapters on oral and manual stimulation. I've found this area to be where women seem to have the least amount of confidence in their sexual ability. If you've been less than secure in this area, you won't be much longer. Here you'll find easy-to-follow instructions on many hand and mouth techniques, the results of which (according to seminar participants nationwide) will blow his mind. For those who enjoy a little whimsy in the bedroom or who have been curious about sexual toys and how to use them, the final chapter of the book was created just for *you*. After reading, you may just find yourself the recipient of a brand new strand of pearls—that is, once he finds out how you intend to *use* them.

It is difficult to adequately capture with words the kind of power you feel from having the ability to put the person you love in total ecstasy. When I say power, I don't mean having power *over* your lover (although men *have* been known to become slaves to Ode to Bryan). I'm talking about a kind of selfless power that comes from *knowing* that you know. Once you are assured of your knowledge, all aspects of your relationship with your husband, lover, or boyfriend will change significantly. As you become physically closer, you'll find the boundaries of your intimacy expanding on every level. There is no greater spiritual exchange between two people than that of lovers loving well.

If I can contribute to furthering this kind of joy in any way, then even on my worst day I've still got the best job in the world.

Chapter Two

Beyond the Bedroom

CREATING YOUR
SENSUAL ENVIRONMENT

*"When I walked into her bedroom, it was like walking
into a fabulous pink boudoir—it was all pink and
glowing and reminded me of her body."*

MALE SEMINAR ATTENDEE,

REAL ESTATE DEVELOPER, AGE 45

Bad Timing, Jilted Feelings

Has this ever happened to you?

You have decided to pull out all the stops and surprise him
with an extravagant romantic dinner, intending to follow it up
with a night of passionate lovemaking. You juggled your schedule, spent a small fortune on exotic fruits, paté, filet mignon,
and a bottle of 1984 Cabernet Sauvignon. You have painstak-
ingly seen to it that no detail has been overlooked.

He arrives home with a pile of work to do and tells you, as
he heads into the kitchen, that all he wants for dinner is a sandwich. You are immediately enraged! You can't believe he's chosen
to work after everything you've done to make the night special.

He can't believe you'd go to so much trouble without checking with him first. What you really feel is rejected. What he really feels is guilty.

In this scenario, it is easier to complain about the time, money, and effort wasted on preparing a beautiful dinner, rather than talk about the rejection you feel because he seems disinterested in a night of romance. But that's where the real hurt lies. The dinner and all the little details involved were just the wrapping on the gift of intimacy. To have that go unaccepted is understandably hurtful.

Unexpected situations come up that curtail even the best of intentions. That's precisely why it's so important to head off disappointments at the pass whenever possible—*especially* when it comes to sex. But the truth is, there is no feeling that sticks with you longer than that of being truly surprised by something wonderful from the person you love.

In this particular case, all it would have taken to avoid hurt feelings was a phone call. Without giving away the surprise you could have just called and said, "Are we still on for dinner?" He then would have had the opportunity to tell you either he couldn't make it because he had to work, or that he only had time for a quick bite. Should *he* have called to inform you about the change in his workload? Sure. But he's only thinking about the crisis at hand. He's not anticipating a problem with you—he has no idea of your surprise. You're the one who has chosen to invest in the big romantic effort. In a case like this, I think it's just good time-management to protect your investment. Besides, had you known about it sooner, you could have devised a Plan B. His sandwich could have been ready when he walked through the door and *you* could have been, too. Knowing you understood his situation, he might have been grateful for a quick sexual stressbuster. On the other hand, if his change of schedule put you out of the mood, you would have an opportunity to make other plans.

When it comes to intimacy and the expression of physical love, there is nothing more exhilarating than complete and total freedom. But total sexual freedom cannot exist unless it's felt by *both* partners. Sometimes a person shuts down sexually because of temporary mood swings but *usually* it's caused by one of these bigger issues: performance anxiety, inexperience, moral boundaries, or body-image.

Secret from Lou's Archives

One of the easiest ways to turn him on is to *not* do what is expected. Don't go for the action spot first—make him wait! Be more like a new lover where he can't anticipate your moves.

Contrary to the very old and inaccurate myth, not all men are ready, willing, and able to have sex at the drop of a hat. Because we've been led to believe this nonsense, we often find ourselves disappointed. There are as many reasons for not being in the mood for sex as there are experiences in a day. It is a mistake to jump to the conclusion that the reason is relationship threatening. The worst thing any of us can do when our partners are out of synch with us sexually is to attempt to pressure them into it. In the first place, it rarely works—and when it does, it often causes our partner to harbor resentment. Why would you even *want* to have to talk someone into making love? That would, after all, defeat the purpose. Obviously, if you find that you and your partner are frequently out of synch sexually, a discussion is warranted. Even then, the problem should be discussed away from the bedroom. Most of the time, however, giving a lover the space to not want sex and not have to feel guilty about it will allow for a much freer exchange the next time the opportunity to make love presents itself.

Of course, when the two of you *do* find yourselves in synch, a little romantic ambiance never hurt anything. And there are times when a subtle hint or two of sexuality have revealed that he's actually more in the mood than he thought he was. There are lots of ways to show him you're feeling amorous other than coming out with a blatant "Let's do it," although that isn't necessarily a bad idea, either. Quite often it takes nothing more than lowering the volume and slowing down the speed of your voice to convey a shift in your intention. You don't want to sound inauthentic, but you do want him to realize there's a change in your agenda. While making casual conversation, speak clearly and enunciate carefully. Whenever you speak with *in*tention, you are more likely to get the *at*tention of your audience.

Secret from Lou's Archives

Men are visual creatures, so consider asking him if he'd like to watch you. If yes, hand him pillows to help prop him up so he has a better view of what you're doing.

If, for some reason, you feel the need to have the suggestion be *his*, there are things you can do to help him suggest it sooner rather than later. Let us not forget, however, manipulation is a practice best left to chiropractors. There is no greater turn-off than to have someone repeatedly refuse your sexual invitations. These ideas are presented in the spirit of sensual communication, assuming that if he knew your intention, he'd find it appealing.

Regardless of what the truth may be, unless it's communicated openly, a refusal of intimacy is almost always *interpreted* by the other person as a lack of desire or waning affection. Because sex is so very revealing both physically and emotionally, there is no escaping the attachment it has to the ego. To offer the most intimate part of yourself, thinking it will be warmly welcomed and exchanged, only to find out it couldn't be *less* welcome, is devastating. In contrast, to reach out sexually and be welcomed is a terrific thing. A couple of weeks after attending one of my seminars, a forty-five-year-old advertising executive from Chicago accompanied her husband to the wedding of his boss's son. As is typical at weddings, where most of us are at least semi-conscious of what the bride and groom are up to after the reception, she and her husband were excited. They left the party, walked down a few hallways, and found a hotel utility closet. Opening the door and pulling her husband inside, the woman pushed her husband against the door and reached for his fly. You can imagine the rest.

Days after the wedding, her husband couldn't stop referring to the "broom closet" episode, as he had dubbed it. The woman told me that it was the sheer spontaneity of the experience that had thrilled him the most.

The perfect romantic setting has its place. On those occasions, it's fun to spend time fussing over an elegant meal, picking out something beautiful to wear, choosing the appropriate music, and generally producing a mood *oozing* with sensuous intention. But you must understand that sensuous intention can just as easily be created from corned beef sandwiches and Budweiser as it can from caviar and Cristal.

The point is that if you're waiting around for candlelight and moonbeams, you could wait yourself right out of the physical urgency that is so much a part of the experience. Mother Nature provided us with hormones for a reason. We are born as sexual beings. Our sexuality creates life and it creates love. It is our most powerful form of communication and is intended for us to use. It does not come with stipulations on how, when, and where to use it.

Many of us get our ideas for romantic encounters from the movies. Unfortunately, in real life we usually don't have access to makeup artists, wardrobe consultants, or set designers. Lovely as these lovemaking scenes are to watch, the filmmakers might think about flashing a disclaimer saying, "Don't try this at home, or you could set yourself up for a major disappointment." If you are trapped inside a photograph of what sensuality is supposed to *look* like, you'll miss out on all the beauty of what sensuality can ultimately *feel* like. *Looks like* is not often the same as *feels like*, and rarely the same as *is*. Feeling sensually aroused comes from within as much as it comes from without.

Reigniting the Flames of Passion

Sometimes in my seminars I hear men and women complaining about couples getting locked into patterns of the same approach, the same position, the same day, the same time, etc. There's no excitement, no butterflies, no danger, no laughter, no anything. First they go a week at a time without sex, then before they even realize it, a whole month has gone by. Pretty soon, so much time has passed that they're both too embarrassed to mention it. All of a sudden they're actually *shy* again with each other.

This situation is not uncommon, yet it is still only representative of a portion of the women I've spoken to about their sex lives. There are other women who keep the rest of the seminar participants on the edge of their seats with wonderful stories of sensual adventures. And don't think for a moment that these stories come only from the young women or women in the first blissful stages of love. Some of the most exciting sensual adventures come from women who have been with the same men for decades. They simply refused to succumb to the sexual boredom that many believe is inevitable to long-term relationships. One couple from Texas, who married in their twenties and are still married after fifteen years, keep a private date night every month: one of them orders from a favorite takeout restaurant, picks up a bottle of wine, and brings it all up to the bedroom, where they spend the rest of the night. As the woman, a psychologist, told me, "Our lives get so fast and busy, there is so little time to slow down and feel like we did when we first got together. In the bedroom, we're halfway to where we want to go."

Another woman and her husband were both married before—he for thirty years, and she for twelve. Knowing they weren't going to reach a twenty-fifth anniversary, they decided to celebrate their marriage every month by doing something special. One of their favorite ways to mark their anniversaries is to dine in the nude. As the woman told me, "We're up to our 115th celebration and they keep getting better!"

You must realize, assuming you're both healthy and that you genuinely care for one another, sexual intensity (or lack thereof) is a personal choice. It's *not* a condition. It can be created or re-created very quickly. The only prerequisites for a truly sensuous and fulfilling sex life for both of you are desire and a little inspiration. The following ideas were conceived and pulled off successfully by women in the seminar in order to stimulate the sexual flow of their relationships. I'm sharing them with you, hoping they might inspire your own creative juices. Remember, your sensual environment belongs to you and your partner. What works for another couple will not necessarily work for the two of you, nor should it. Yet sometimes, stepping outside those boundaries of the sexual box you're accustomed to is exactly what it takes to *re*ignite the flames of passion.

For her husband's thirty-fifth birthday, a housewife from a suburb outside of New York City decided to greet him with a little surprise when he'd returned home after being out of town on business for several days. When he entered the front door, he found a note waiting for him on the foyer table. It read, "Happy Birthday Darling, Follow Directions Explicitly: turn up the heat to 85; totally disrobe; put on the David Sanborn CD; and sit in the Eames chair [which was covered with a towel]; blindfold yourself, and don't say a word. When you are ready, clap your hands." At which point, the woman came into the room and proceeded to massage him with warm oil and feed him olives, grapes, and apricots. Then she did a hot/cold shift with her mouth (see Chapter 7) while performing oral sex. "My husband told me it was the most amazing sensation experience he'd ever experienced. And it totally revved up our sex life."

Another woman, in her mid-forties and from Los Angeles, recounted this story: "I had been taking a class in signing for the deaf, so my husband had been used to me being gone every Tuesday and Thursday evening. So the night of The Sexuality Seminar I told him a white lie and said I had a special study class for signing. The next morning, I called him and confessed that I really hadn't been at my regular class the night before, but I'd gone to The Sexuality Seminar instead. At first he didn't believe me. Then I said 'Meet me at home, be nude, and I'll prove it to you.'" He did and she told me that it was one of the best afternoons of lovemaking they'd had since they'd gotten married.

Yet another woman, after going through their usual weekend

argument about what movie to rent, acquiesced to her husband, agreeing to forgo her love story for his action adventure. Later, at the video store, she had an idea. She walked out a little while later with both the action adventure *and* a pornographic film. She put the porn film in the action adventure case and handed it to him, saying she would make them some popcorn and be right in. Instead of going to the kitchen, she went to the bedroom and put on one of his shirts, a sexy bra, and a thong. Then she joined him in front of the television. As it turned out, he got his action adventure, after all.

An elegant middle-aged woman told me of accompanying her lover, an older, very regal gentleman in his mid-sixties, to the Jockey Club in New York for lunch. It was late afternoon and the club's restaurant was virtually empty except for one other couple across the room. Under the circumstances, they were both surprised by how little attention they were receiving from the waiter. After bringing them some wine, the waiter had left them alone for a long time. She could see that her partner was starting to become impatient with the lack of service, in spite of the fact they were in no hurry at all. She wondered why he always had to get so uptight in restaurants. Knowing that an unpleasant scene was imminent, she reached under the table in their booth. Putting her hand on his crotch, she began to rub it gently, increasing the intensity as his attention obviously shifted from the missing waiter. He was shocked at her boldness, but couldn't stop himself from reacting to it. *She* was surprised at her behavior, too, as it was rare for her to be the aggressor in any of their sexual encounters. For some reason, it excited her beyond belief to have been able to squelch his anger with her bare hand, and she felt giddy with excitement. She unzipped his fly, freed his penis and continued working on him. As he grabbed the napkin and rushed it under the table, the only thing he could muster was, "*God*, I hope that waiter doesn't come back now!" To this day, he has never complained about having to wait for service in a restaurant again. A warning: *If you should try this yourself*, do *make sure that the tablecloth reaches at least halfway to the floor.*

Secret from Lou's Archives

Women and men have distinctly different scents. Men tend to smell muskier, and women sweeter. There are also different scents among the different races: my sources tell me that Caucasian, African-American, and Asian men all have distinct body scents.

In another scenario, a nurse from Toronto changed her husband's expectation of Christmas forever. In his stocking, she put several "gift certificates" entitling him to particular sexual requests. He could ask for anything he wanted from her sexually. A week or so after Christmas, she came home and there, at the top of the stairs, was her husband wearing nothing but a smile and a certificate. After fifteen years of marriage, the ritual continues and this couple *insists* that their sex drive, their commitment, and their love for each other has only gotten stronger.

More Ways to Steam Things Up
- Talk explicitly about what you want to do to him, and he to you, in bed. This can be thrilling to a man— especially when you never use that kind of language outside of bed. Practice in front of a mirror to see what you'll look like if you're unsure.

- Tell him discreetly that you're wearing sexy, skimpy, or no lingerie at all, while the rest of world sees you dressed classically; this will usually please him far more than putting your sex appeal on display. Every man loves the idea of bringing out the wild side of a woman. *Believing he alone has the capacity to do that creates a bond unlike any other.* It's not just sensual—it's mental, emotional, and spiritual as well.

- Call him at work, where he cannot respond (in action) to what you're saying or suggesting. This is another form of foreplay that helps build the sexual tension and heighten the anticipation of your next meeting.

Bodily Bliss

I've had conversations with men of every age, race, location, and income level about what they feel to be the single most significant element in defining an incredible sexual experience with a woman. Nary a one of them has differed in his perspective on this issue. It isn't a perfect figure. It isn't physical beauty. It isn't even expertise.

Because of the way we've been conditioned socially, it might be difficult to believe, but it is true: what men want more than anything else is simply for us to be *into* it. During an intimate encounter, a man is looking for your mind, body, and soul to be in full relationship with the project at hand. He wants to know beyond a shadow of a doubt that he turns you on, and that there's no place else in the world you'd rather be than with him, making love.

In the same way, men love body language. They respond to a

body that is totally committed to whatever it's doing. Whether you're eating, playing sports, telling a story, or kissing doesn't matter. If you're committed, men notice. That's why it's important, when sex is on your mind, to make sure your body is reflecting that message. This doesn't mean to stand or move provocatively. Overkill isn't necessary either. But you don't want to appear *un*sure about something you *are* sure about. Extend yourself, rather than close up. Stretch, stand tall, and move freely. Let him know you are in touch with your body and that you are absolutely aware of what you're doing.

At the same time, you don't want to stage or exaggerate your intentions. A forty-three-year-old male paper broker told me of his recent visit to his very posh gym. As he was using the bench press, he happened to catch sight of a woman in a formfitting aerobics outfit, stretching on the railing above him. He soon realized that she was not wearing any underwear; no thong, no Calvin Kleins, nothing. Instead of being turned on by such an obvious display of her body, he was actually turned off. "It was just too brazen, too overt, too trying-too-hard. It's much sexier for me to see a woman enjoying herself, totally immersed in what she is doing—whatever she's wearing."

The reason this is such valuable information is that women tend to be more inhibited sexually by the appearance of their own bodies than anything else. To attempt to hide, cover up, or camouflage an imperfection in your stomach, butt, breasts, or thighs during sex is not only a waste of time, it is a waste of your energy. In the first place, he's either going to see it or feel it anyway, especially if you're going out of your way to make sure he doesn't. And in the second place, chances are he doesn't care.

Be aware of the sensuality in everything you see, feel, touch, taste, and smell. He will not only respond to your sensory awakening, chances are he'll want to be a part of the experience. For example, a lawyer recently shared a story about a night she went to a nightclub with some friends after work. She was wearing a suit and a pair of low pumps. While listening to the music, she very consciously played with her shoe, letting it dangle on the ends of her toes. A short time later, a man who had been sitting at the table next to hers came over and gently tapped her on the shoulder, and said, "I am very sorry to interrupt you, but I'm afraid you're either going to have to stop doing that with your foot, or knowingly continue to drive me crazy."

What was interesting is that he didn't continue to make conversation; in fact, he left almost immediately. The woman wasn't wearing what one would call a sexy outfit, nor could he even see her face from where he sat. What turned him on was the sheer consciousness with which she twirled her shoe. To him, that reeked of sensuality. I've come to find out that many men feel the same way. We're so often completely unaware of how the simplest of gestures affect those who are watching us.

Secret from Lou's Archives

However demure men may want us to appear in public, they want us unrestrained in private. In fact, it's precisely this dichotomy that drives them wild. The more collected our public persona, the more unrestrained our private one can be.

Don't get me wrong. I'm not going to tell you you're mistaken about men being visual creatures. They are typically much more so than us. But their desire for, and even sometimes preoccupation with, the perfect female body takes place *before* the sexual encounter. Once you're there, the only thing that really matters about your body to them is that it expresses a willingness to thoroughly and freely enjoy the experience. While making love with an enthusiastic partner, men don't have the wherewithal to focus on imperfections, because they perceive what they have as perfect.

Feeling Beautiful: It's Up to You

In spite of the knowledge that your free sensual spirit will have *him* thinking you're beautiful, what ultimately matters most is how *you* feel about yourself. It is only appropriate to dress or act a certain way to please your man when it's your choice—and if, in so doing, you derive at least as much pleasure for yourself. If garter belts, thongs, and teddies aren't your style, don't wear them, and don't be fooled into thinking the stereotypical picture of a woman in black lace and heels is the only one that works. I know many men who think otherwise.

One man, a lawyer from Boston, told me that what gets him most excited is when his wife (a history professor) puts on his boxer shorts and tank top. "When she's wearing that outfit, I go crazy!" In fact, I have it on very good authority that when women wear jeans and a T-shirt it is every bit as much a turn-on for some men as a garter belt and push-up bra. I've even known men who simply cannot *resist* a woman in soft flannel pajamas. Above all else, you need to be comfortable with your presentation. Your comfort, both in mind and body, is the key to your sexual freedom.

The only thing you both *have to be* in bed is clean. None of us should have to be subjected to a sexual partner who isn't. I'm not just talking about your private parts. I can't tell you how regularly this comes up in both the men's and women's seminars. Hair, ears, fingernails, toenails, and feet are often overlooked and left unscrubbed in the haste to get into bed. I would never have felt the need to state the obvious in a book like this if didn't come up in nearly every seminar. Evidently, we tend to assume that we all groom ourselves in the same way. Also, we are horrified at the thought of discussing the subject: to tell a lover that you are turned off by his lack of cleanliness is uncomfortable for both of you. But there is no excuse for having to feel "dirtied" by someone with whom you're going to be intimate. Anyone willing to share himself or herself in this manner deserves a partner who is well groomed. If you're too tired for another shower or bath, you're too tired for sex.

And while we're on the subject of cleanliness, I just want to mention a word about the natural odor of the human body. I understand that some men and women prefer to go au naturel and not wear deodorant, but I think you're taking a risk here. Let me recount a story of a successful businessman in his early sixties, trim and quite the gentleman. He had been with a woman who was in her late forties and was very much attracted to her: she was fit, active, and fun-loving—all qualities he appreciated and admired. After the second or third sexual encounter, he became unavoidably aware of her bad body odor. He felt very awkward bringing this up, as they didn't know each other *that* well yet, but he felt really turned off. Need I say more? I think it's a shame to go through all the emotional stages involved in becoming ready for physical intimacy only to discover, once you get down to the bare essentials, that you can't stomach the way your lover smells. And through scores of interviews, I've found that the biggest offenders are the most oblivious to it. What I suggest is that if you lead even a moderately active lifestyle, experience any level of stress, or sweat for any reason, and don't use deodorant, in spite of the fact that you shower daily, you are a candidate for body odor. Bathing is essential, of course. But if it were enough, deodorant would not have been invented.

Ambience

Don't despair, you don't have to be Michelangelo to come up with creative ideas to add sparks to your lovemaking. There is nothing more exhilarating than being creative about how to love. You and your partner must decide, based on your individual personal styles, what whets your appetites. The secret to your success is *not* to do what he would expect, but to step outside the box and go to a place you've never been before.

Secret from Lou's Archives

TV is the biggest robber of intimacy because it draws your attention out of the room and away from the person you're with. If you want to keep your partner's attention available, try quieter activities, like reading or listening to music.

A sensual environment is not limited to the bedroom and can be *any* environment where the two of you are inspired to engage in sexual activity. Candlelight, a roaring fire, fine champagne, and soft music are lovely touches, of course. But if that's the *only* type of scene that inspires your libido, you may find yourself waiting an awfully long time between sexual encounters. Remember, unlike our male counterparts, the longer we women go without an orgasm, the longer we usually *can* go without one. And the more often we have them, the more often it seems we *want* them. While I haven't seen this phenomenon documented scientifically, it's no secret that the longer men go without a release, the more intense their need to have one becomes.

Power of Lights

Men are visual creatures and they will respond to visual cues. So ladies, don't think you're alone in believing that soft lighting is synonymous with romance. In the movies, rare is the love scene that doesn't take place in front of the fire, surrounded by candlelight, in the glow of a sunset, under twinkling stars, or during the innocence of daybreak. Thanks to modern technology, the association between dim lights and love is deeply ingrained in the human psyche. But let's be honest, the sensuous effects of firelight date as far back as the Stone Age. Hollywood simply knew a good thing when they heard about it and embellished on a concept that already worked.

The most obvious benefit of soft lighting is the change in mood it automatically elicits. Our voices become lower, enticing us to move nearer to each other and requiring us to listen more carefully. These small details—gentle conversation, closer physical contact, and the willingness to hear what someone else is saying—are very important steps on the path to romance.

But mood isn't the only element of romance affected positively by the dimming of the lights. Let's face it, soft lighting has an aesthetic value as well. It is very kind to lines, bags, blemishes, and other pesky facial flaws that are best not displayed under flourescent lights. Any light coming from behind you, rather than from in front or above you, is going to be more flattering to your entire presentation. Referred to in the film industry and in photography as backlighting, it is often used to take years off the faces of models and celebrities. I must say, it doesn't do any harm to the rest of the body either. Cellulite and love handles also seem to be upstaged by backlight. I often recommend to seminar attendees to, when preparing for a nighttime tryst where moonlight isn't available, use low-wattage colored lightbulbs, which now come in a variety of shades and can be found almost anywhere regular bulbs are sold. The pink or peach shades not only provide the advantage of low light, they also add a beautiful hue to your skin tone, much the same as a sunrise or sunset would do.

CANDLES

While not all of us have a fireplace to fill a room with soft, warm light, candles are entirely practical and inexpensive, too. Depending on the size of the room, it can take one, two, or three candles to give your love nest an ethereal, transportive glow.

Types of Candles (by no means an exhaustive list)

- Spice: sage, cedar, rosemary, lavender, vanilla

- Fruit: pear, orange, peach, blueberry, bayberry, lemon

- Flower: gardenia, rose, tuberose, jasmine

- Essential Oils: patchouli, musk

Tips on Candles

- Orange- or citrus-scented candles are popular among men.

- Ylang-ylang scents are considered aphrodisiacs.

- It's best not to combine floral with fruit scents.

- If you're unsure of how he may react, try a vanilla-scented candle, which is very mild.

- Don't use a heavily scented candle at dinner; it will interfere with the taste of the food.

- Never leave candles unattended.

- Put a small amount of water in the bottom of a votive candle holder; this will automatically extinguish the candle in case you should forget to blow it out, preventing the holder from becoming so hot it might shatter.

Soft light provides a psychological advantage for those who may feel uncomfortable about a sexual encounter, or shy in the first few interludes with a brand new lover. Regardless of how right lovemaking may feel emotionally, whenever you're trying something different sexually—be it a new partner, position, or sexual act—it is natural to be nervous. Sometimes, a little less light on the subject can help to minimize your self-consciousness.

When you're creating a sensual environment, remember that it belongs to both of you. Always give yourselves the freedom to just say no to sex, but also remember that part of love is to be there for each other sometimes even when you'd rather be somewhere else. No one feels like making love all the time. Still, it is often those times when you least expect it that sex is the most exciting. Whether it is slow, romantic sex or quick and raunchy, when you're with someone whom you care deeply about, it is *always* making love.

Chapter Three

The Art of Kissing

A KISS IS NEVER
JUST A KISS

*"I'd always hated the way my husband kissed
yet I didn't know how to show him how I wanted him
to really kiss me. I couldn't believe the simple
and loving technique you taught me to show him."*

FEMALE SEMINAR ATTENDEE,

NEW YORK STOCKBROKER, AGE 36

Kissing is where all sexual synergy starts. When your lips touch another's, it's the first sign, the first taste, of what is to come. At the same time, despite your mutual attraction to one another, if a kiss feels "off," it's difficult to not feel turned off. A married woman in a seminar told me that she doesn't like the way her husband kisses. I asked, "Then how can you go beyond that if you don't like to kiss?" She said, "We just don't kiss; we skip that part."

I say, What a shame. Kissing is one of the best ways to get all the juices flowing. But as I listened to countless other women, I began to hear similar stories about their so-called "kissing dissatisfaction." Since then I have heard a number of women and men in my seminars describe their disappointment that kissing is no longer a part of their sexual relationships.

Most of the time, they talk about how passionate their kisses *used* to be, when they lasted for hours and were the driving force for every sexual encounter. But over time, that passion has slipped away from them, and the kisses slowly decrease in both quantity and intensity. Exactly when the passion began to fade is never quite clear, but most women are at a loss as to how or *if* it can be regained.

The good news is that the disappointment is not specific to men or women, but women tend to volunteer their feelings of disappointment, and men won't bring it up unless asked. But the fact remains, when kisses lose their heat, it is missed by both of you.

Don't be under the misconception that he's no longer interested in kissing you passionately. He may not be interested in talking about it, because men are not often comfortable in any discussion that allows their vulnerability to be seen. What men want is evidence that they turn you on. More than anything else, that's what turns *them* on. You can send that message in no uncertain terms by the way you kiss him.

Secret from Lou's Archives

Men will often watch how a woman eats and drinks to get a sense of how she will kiss and make love. The more robust a woman's appetite, the more likely she'll be open and passionate.

What is sadder than those who say they've lost the passion are the confessions from those who say they've never had it. To be spending time in a romantic relationship without experiencing the ride of a passionate kiss is unconscionable. Kissing is the essence of romance out of which passion emerges, and in an ongoing relationship, you deserve sensuality. Whether you're trying to create it or re-create it doesn't matter. No one else is more entitled to passion, regardless of age or length of time in a relationship, than you are. The only prerequisite for passion is a desire to have it.

The History of Kissing

Kissing just *may* be the greatest form of communication ever invented. According to one legend, the kiss was created by medieval knights for the ridiculous purpose of determining whether their wives had been nipping at the mead barrel while they were off crusading. Fortunately, kissing did not remain limited to alcohol detection. In the past, some young women believed babies were the result of a passionate kiss. (They had the right idea, of course, but they just didn't follow the thought to its biological conclusion.) Indeed, kissing not only survived, it has thrived, and for good reason.

Secret from Lou's Archives

The word "kiss" comes from the 12th-century English word "cyssan," which refers to "wet, soul, or tongue."

The more likely (and sweeter) explanation of the origin of the kiss extends back to the bond between mother and child when, before the invention of jars of baby food, mothers had to first chew food in order to give it to their child. The emotional connection that takes place here goes way beyond the giving and receiving of food. It's about peace and safety and a sensation of being exactly where each other belongs. The reason a baby often falls asleep at her mother's breast long after she's finished eating is that the feeling of lips on flesh is so comforting.

Human lips not only contain sebaceous glands, they also are filled with extremely sensitive nerve endings. When these nerve endings come in contact with another person's lips or skin, the connection creates a language of its own. We all want to be fluent in lip language in order to send clear messages or receive them in the spirit with which they are intended. A kiss can be kind, empathetic, sympathetic, sad, final, cute, polite, invitational, passionate, ravaging, or aloof. If a picture is worth a thousand words, then a kiss is worth a billion. It can be used to deliver any kind of communication one desires, provided one is skilled in the art. And no kiss has ever been wasted—not even the kiss of death.

For our purposes, however, I'm going to focus on those kisses given and received with the sole intention of stirring the embers of passion—before, during, and after lovemaking. It should never be forgotten that when it comes to romance, there are few tools available to us more powerful than the kiss. For that reason, you must be mindful of every kiss you give and every kiss you receive. Kisses send messages—especially in romance. Being mindful of your kisses simply means to be aware of the language that is spoken at all times and to never allow your lips to speak anything other than the truth. And although kissing, just like loving, comes to us instinctively, both benefit greatly from instruction and practice.

That Tingling Feeling

In spite of what your darling mother may have told you, a "fresh" mouth is a *good* thing. If it sounds remedial to say that your mouth and breath should be clean before kissing, forgive me for stating the obvious. But we've all been in situations where either our partner's breath isn't nearly as desirable as he is, or we can sense that ours isn't. And it's not just breath. Food that has, for some reason, decided to remain outside the mouth, rather than join the rest of the party inside, may leave deleterious leftovers. That rebellious piece of spinach, that flamboyant bit of caviar, or the lone black bean that insists on making a spectacle of itself by adhering to your or his front-most tooth may also be a culprit. It's not the least bit cute and can be a real mood killer.

But bad breath and food stuck in our teeth can happen to the best of us, and when they do, the only way to handle them is with kindness and humor, removing them as quickly as possible. No one should be made to feel badly about being human. On the other hand, if your lover's breath is a bit offensive—*say* something. I know you wouldn't consider kissing somebody who didn't care if he offended you, so help him out. And be gracious when he does the same for you. These little problems are easy to fix and any momentary embarrassment can be quelled with, "And now my dear, you are perfect . . . once again."

The following is a list of tips and suggestions I've picked up from clients on how to remedy or prevent these potential kiss stoppers:

- When brushing your teeth, don't forget to brush your tongue and the roof of your mouth. They are the repositories of bad-breath germs and must be swept clean. Brushing these areas will keep your breath fresher for much longer.

- Collect those little bottles of mouthwash you get in hotels and keep one in every purse. You can also purchase them in grocery and drugstores where they display travel and trial-size products.

- Never leave home without mints.

- Keep mints in a little box by the side of your bed. They're great for eliminating morning breath.

- When one of you eats spicy or strong foods, such as garlic or onion, you both should eat some. The smell isn't nearly as offensive when you've both consumed the same food, as your chemistries are better matched.

- Parsley is a great odor eater, so if it arrives as a garnish on your plate at a restaurant, take advantage of it. And don't forget to pick up a bunch at the grocery store when you're doing the cooking.

- If your lover's breath doesn't smell fresh, take a mint for yourself, and *then* offer one to him.

- Dental tape is three times more effective than dental floss. Keep a roll in your purse. If you're going to be somewhere without a purse, put a piece of tape in your bra or pocket. (Never use it while other people are watching.)

- An Oolit is a fairly new little gadget. It is a flexible, serrated plastic strip, used to scrape the entire tongue in order to remove odor-causing bacteria that remains on the tongue after brushing. You'll be amazed to find out what lingers there.

- Make a deal with your lover right from the get-go to do a quick check of each other's teeth upon completion of your meals for food that doesn't belong there.

- Delicately touch your napkin to the sides of your mouth after every few bites, whether you think there's anything there or not—just to be safe. That is precisely what napkins are for.

- If you see that your lover has a crumb or drop of something on his face or mouth, take your napkin and gently wipe it away. If you're not within comfortable wiping distance, tell him about it in a soft voice or give him a discreet little signal to wipe his mouth.

- Excuse yourself to freshen up on your way out of a restaurant. It will give him an opportunity to do the same. At home, mention casually that you need to freshen up; make sure you have mouthwash and dental tape out where it can be seen so he doesn't have to look through your drawers or cabinets in order to make himself presentable.

Lips Are Not Just for Kissing

I want to share a story with you about men and lips. For years one of my dearest male friends and I have volunteered on the AIDS ward at a Los Angeles hospital. Whenever possible, we would synchronize our breaks in order to get a snack together. During the summer months we usually opted for an ice cream cone. I remember once, fairly early on in our friendship, we were sitting outside eating our cones when he looked over and said, "Lou, you're gonna have to finish that up pretty quickly or this table we're sitting at is going to start rising off the ground." Knowing he didn't mean any harm, I burst into laughter and asked him why. He told me that men have a real thing about women and cones. Evidently ladies, whenever a man eyes a woman licking an ice cream cone, he imagines her doing the same thing to his penis.

Several weeks later, we were driving in his car when we saw a girl crossing the street, licking and sucking on a cone, oblivious to anything else. My friend told me to watch the way the men around were looking. I was shocked. Every man at the intersection, as well as those stopped in their cars at the light, was mesmerized by this woman. They couldn't keep their eyes off her mouth! "Lou, let me tell you something," my friend said. "If there is a woman crossing the street eating an ice cream cone, she'll stop traffic."

A professional woman from Florida told me this similar story. Not too long ago she and her boyfriend were getting ready to go out somewhere. She was doing a bit of last minute primping with lipstick while he waited patiently. She said something like, "Just trying to make them pretty so you'll want to kiss them, dear." He let out a laugh and said, "Kissing isn't exactly what I had in mind." As it turns out, it is also common knowledge among men that when they look at women's lips and find them appealing, they don't necessarily think about what we'd be like to kiss. And ladies, men have shared with me that they respond this way when watching a female newscaster. More than likely, their minds are focused on our lips touching something located further south on their bodies.

Getting in Sync

At no other time is there more intention while kissing than during a romantic prelude. The key, as we discussed in Chapter 2, is to make that intention *yours*. Kissing is the beginning, middle, and end of incredible lovemaking. For that reason, its power should never be underestimated. If you and your lover are not connected to one another's kisses, there will always be limits to your passion. In order for your sexual spirits to be set free, it is absolutely essential that you kiss and be kissed in a manner that creates heat. An advertising executive from Chicago put it this way: "My boyfriend is a hot, hot kisser. A few minutes of that and I am ready. When he's on top of me and deeply inside, I feel his breath, his hot chest, and we're kissing—I feel loved, lusted for, and safe."

Kissing, like so many elements of romance, is subjective. What one person likes isn't necessarily going to have the same effect on somebody else. That's very often the root of the trouble. A kiss that may have driven a previous lover crazy with desire could be turning your current lover off completely. It isn't that he doesn't like to kiss, he just may not like to be kissed that *way*. Obviously, the same applies to you. If his kisses are turning you off, or leaving you less than turned on, it's a problem. The solution, however, is not as difficult as it seems. What doesn't work is to tell him his kisses don't do it for you. Need I mention the fragility of the male ego? What *also* doesn't work is to say and do nothing about the problem. If you don't let him know you need something different, he's not likely to give it to you.

> *Secret from Lou's Archives*
> The most important thing you can do for your lips is to keep them soft and clean. A makeup artist I know recommends eye cream, as it absorbs better than regular lip salve.

SHOW HIM HOW

The way to address the so-called "kissing problem" is to show him how you like to be kissed. By following these four steps, you could have your perfect kiss as early as tonight:

1. Tell him how much you love to kiss.

2. Kiss him the way you love to be kissed so he knows exactly what that feels like.

3. Stop, pull back, and say to him, "Will you show me how it feels to be kissed by me?"

4. If he kisses you right, make sure he knows how much you enjoyed it and show him how very stimulated you feel. Men tend not to forget what gets them results. (If he didn't do it right, repeat steps 1–3 as many times as necessary.)

Leave Him Breathless

In spite of how differently each of us wants to be kissed, there are a few things I've heard over and over again from both men and women that bear repeating. These are tried-and-true techniques guaranteed to give you and your partner a great kiss:

- Tight, closed lips are not associated with passion. No one likes to kiss a dead fish. If you really don't want to kiss, it's better not to do it at all than to do it without feeling.

- When your lips touch his skin, he should be able to feel the *inside* rim of your lips, not just the outside. You can see what a difference this makes if you try it on your own hand.

- Add your tongue intermittently at first, gradually increasing its involvement in each kiss. When kissing, make sure your tongue is not moving in and out of your mouth so quickly that it resembles a woodpecker. This is NOT a turn-on.

- Men love to be kissed, nibbled, and nuzzled, but again, it's important to move slowly and explore every inch of his body like a newfound treasure.

- Pretend you just finished brushing your teeth. Run your tongue along your teeth and gum lines as if you were checking to make sure they're clean and smooth. Do the exact same thing in his mouth while kissing (although you'll be using the underside of your tongue to do it), and see what kind of a reaction you get.

- As things start to heat up and you move on to other elements of foreplay, you are likely to find yourself far from his lips. The lips are home base to sensuality, and wherever you roam, remember to go home. Think of kissing his lips as gunning his sexual engine. You need to keep it revved up.

- GO SLOWLY. The more excited he gets, the faster he'll want to go. But don't forget it is these slow, mindful moves that got him excited to begin with. Don't rush or let him rush you.

These tips are obviously best used during a long, romantic encounter. Fast, urgent sex can be as hot as sex that lasts for hours, and the rush of skipping the foreplay can be a total turn-on. But a slow buildup of intensity through kissing can create that inexplicable synergy between you and your lover that, once experienced, will always remain.

Secret from Lou's Archives

The man who doesn't like a tongue in his ear is rare, but the woman who does is rarer still.

Kissing Hot Spots
- Earlobes
- Bellybuttons (you can tongue him here or suck as well)
- Nipples, nipples, nipples
- Toes and fingers

- Backs of his knees

- Base of his neck

- Crook of his arm

- Small of his back

- Any area that rarely sees sunshine or is usually covered by clothes

The Swirl

Along with kissing, The Swirl is an outstanding way to rev up your man's engine. The idea was a result of a man who said, "Most men are only aware of a thin column down their bodies—we think, eat, feel, have sex, etc., but we ignore the other areas of our bodies. Like the arms and our backs. Let women know we are dying to have them woken up—we just ignore them."

Your partner will typically touch you the way he likes to be touched. For most men that tends to be a firm, direct touch to action spots. Women tend to touch more lightly and more tentatively. This makes sense as men's skin is thicker and denser than ours. To see how this feels try it on your own leg first—you'll need your leg as you'll be using both hands so your arm won't work.

Step A: On the bare skin of your thigh, lightly scratch, using your nails, from your knee to your pubic hair in a straight line. Adjust pressure to your preference.

Step B: Now, scratching over the same area, use a large wavy motion—be sure they are generous waves.

In step A, what you'll likely feel (as will he) are the little nerves saying, "Oh, goodie, I'm next." In step B, your nerves will be saying, "Oh, my God, I hope I'm next."

This can be done on any area of his body; legs, arms, head, neck—you choose. And, of course, lightly on his genitals.

The best part is it can be done in public, obviously in a reserved form, with others being none the wiser.

Secret from Lou's Archives

When French or soul kissing, be careful to avoid two things: 1) sucking too hard on his tongue; 2) making your tongue too pointy. Apparently it feels like kissing Woody Woodpecker.

Types of Kisses

- THE FRENCH KISS (OR SOUL KISSING). Although tongue kissing is known in many cultures, the naming of this activity as a French Kiss is apparently from the British and Americans who attributed anything sexually liberated to the French. This is by far the most widely known kind of kiss. A good French kiss can last for hours. Indeed, I know of a contest in which a couple kissed for a straight twenty-four hours! Here, rhythm is everything. You need to alternate the rhythm, suck on his tongue, and move your tongue around.

- THE ESKIMO KISS. This is really an olfactory kiss, preferable to other types of kisses in certain cultures. In an Eskimo kiss you rub cheek to cheek, or nose to nose, taking in each other's scent.

- THE EYELASH KISS (BUTTERFLY KISS). This one's a very popular parent-to-child kiss. Your eyelashes are fluttered rapidly on the chosen body part—cheeks, lips, nipples. But one woman has remarked, "I love to catch my eyelashes on his chest hair."

- THE DANCING KISS. This is a version of the Eskimo, cheek-to-cheek kiss, a quick embrace that you and your partner can do in the presence of others.

- THE PROPRIETARY KISS. This is the type that your partner plants on you after you've been talking to that charming gentleman for over twenty minutes.

- THE HAND KISS. This is a truly seductive move if done by the right man. Allowing his lips to linger on the inner part of your palm can certainly catch your interest.

- THE LIP SUCKING KISS. Suck on the bottom part of your partner's lip and enjoy its full fleshiness. Avoid the upper lip: this may cause discomfort!

- HICKEYS. Hickeys are usually an indication that someone is still in school, yet I am sure we all have one or two in our pasts: the reddish-brown bruises on our necks left by sucking are hard to forget.

The Subtleties of Kissing

If you were to keep score of all the kisses exchanged between you and your lover, no doubt you would discover that subtle kisses, as a rule, win more points than bold kisses. There is nothing more romantic than being taken by surprise with a short but meaningful little kiss on the back of the neck, the forehead, the nose, or the eyelids at a time when you least expect it. It is lovely to be interrupted while engaged in nonsexual activities such as working, watching television, gardening, grocery shopping, dancing, dining, housecleaning, or cooking with a brief reminder that you are loved. These special kisses are not only fun to give and receive, they also aren't as offensive to those who happen to be watching as so many public displays of affection are.

The kiss that should *never* be overlooked, however, is the after kiss. Whether you've just spent an entire evening of passionate lovemaking or five minutes in the bathroom on an airplane, when the sex part is over, there must be an exchange of at least one sweet kiss. It can be planted on the lips, the cheek, the nose, the forehead, or the eyelid, but this tender after kiss is an expression of love. It may last only a mere second, yet it speaks volumes.

From Post Office to Spin the Bottle, kissing games have long been considered romantic folderol. Here is a game that came up once in a seminar that has been played to the satisfaction of many. Both the kisser and the kissee begin with their eyes closed. It is the kisser's job to plant a kiss on the lips of the kissee without making skin contact anywhere else *other* than the kissee's lips. This game may sound easy, but you will be surprised how often a nose, cheek, or eye gets in the way. After a little practice, however, you will begin to feel the heat radiating off each other's faces and become aware of which facial features produce different types of warmth.

There is no reason in the world why anyone should have to miss out on the pleasure of great sensual kissing. To kiss with abandon is to kiss freely and communicate all the subtlety and range of your feelings.

Chapter Four

Safety Is Essensual

*"There is no one more capable or responsible
for taking care of you than you."*

LOU PAGET

Dispelling the Myths

My purpose here is not merely to provide you with information
to help you be better in bed. The ultimate goal for all of us is to
be *smarter* in bed. Mastering technique is just a small piece of
the bigger picture. Knowing this information is one thing,
knowing how to negotiate is another tool for safe sex. Admittedly,
a chapter on the precautions and risk factors involved in sexual
intimacy isn't as tantalizing as some of the other chapters might
be. I would, however, advise you to read this one in its entirety
before passing judgment. There *is* a little gem in store for you,
and I guarantee you'll be eternally grateful, and so will your
lover. Besides, it would be irresponsible of me, or anyone else,
to offer advice on sexual interaction without discussing safety.
These days, safety is essential. And I happen to think safe sex
can also be es*sensual*.

Sex is often considered something cheap and dirty and
immoral—especially for women. Sex isn't any of those things.
Regardless of anyone's religious or moral beliefs, sex itself is not

bad. We either have sex or end the human race. When, where, how, and with whom we have sex are individual choices. The *only* two things that ever make sex *wrong* is if it's entered into without absolute respect for ourselves and our partners, or without a full understanding of the possible consequences. We're talking about a life-creating, life-altering, and in some cases, life-ending act. I can't think of anything *more* worthy of our respect and understanding.

It wasn't too long ago that the term "safe sex" referred strictly to being kept safe from an unwanted pregnancy. Today when we hear the term, we immediately think of AIDS. There is no question that HIV (*h*uman *i*mmunodeficiency *v*irus) and AIDS (*a*cquired *i*mmuno*d*eficiency *s*yndrome) deserve every bit of the attention that they have received. AIDS can not only kill, but often strips people of all their hope, dignity, and quality of life in the process.

However, there are several problems with thinking that safe sex is only necessary for protection against AIDS. First, since the media and the population at large tend to associate AIDS with homosexuality and intravenous drug use, and most of us do not fall into either category, we tend to distance ourselves from the very real risk of contracting HIV or AIDS. The fact is, the fastest growing risk groups for contracting HIV in the U.S. are straight women and their children. Furthermore, we tend to restrict our awareness of safe sex to the threat of AIDS when there are several very potent and dangerous sexually transmitted diseases (STDs) spreading rampantly, some of which are equally as life-threatening. I think we can all agree: a person who dies of cervical cancer or hepatitis isn't any *less* dead than a person who dies from AIDS-related complications.

We have too much information easily available to be irresponsible about sex. Anyone unwilling to ensure his or her safety before entering a sexual relationship has no business being in one. There is nothing unkind, implied or otherwise, about insisting on safe sex until you know beyond a doubt that each of you is healthy. Quite the contrary, it should be considered a display of honor. If you don't honor your health and well being, why would he? By the same token, if he's not willing to honor his health and well being, why would you?

Secret from Lou's Archives

Many women develop bladder or vaginal infections when they become sexually active with a new partner. This is not at all surprising: you are introducing into the vagina new organisms from your partner's condom, semen, and skin and your body needs time to adjust.

I know a woman, Elena, who, when she asked her potential lover if he had been tested, assured her that he had and that the test result was negative. Yet six months into their relationship, on the weekend they were moving in together, Elena was hospitalized with severe pulmonary distress and quickly diagnosed with HIV infection. In spite of what her boyfriend had told her, she learned that he had been positive for over two years and had infected both his ex-wife and a former girlfriend, in addition to Elena.

You can't be too cautious.

Finally, after all this time, and all the different ways to prevent them, unwanted pregnancies are still on the rise in this country. What this tells us is that as we become more sexual, we're also becoming less responsible, and there is simply no excuse for this neglect. Regardless of the fact that we can and should enjoy sex for other reasons besides procreation, anything serving such an important function should command the utmost respect from all of us. Mother Nature could have just as easily had us become pregnant by eating a certain kind of fruit or taking a certain type of pill. But she chose the intimacy of sexual relations as the way to propagate the species, and that's something we should never take for granted.

The Facts About STDs

Sexually transmitted diseases (STDs) can be contracted by anyone having unprotected sex. As a thirty-four-year-old woman said, "Hey, even though I've only been with low mileage guys, there's still a risk." You are not immune by virtue of your age, ethnicity, education, profession, or socioeconomic status. In fact, one in every fifteen Americans will contract a sexually transmitted disease this year and one in four Americans already has one. What further complicates matters is the fact that it is often difficult to tell who has an STD; many people who are infected look and feel fine and can be blissfully unaware they are infected. For women especially, many STDs have no obvious symptoms until there is already irreparable damage (this is true of chlamydia, which I discuss below). Quite often women are not given the tragic news until they want to start a family and learn that an asymptomatic STD has robbed them of that right, unless they resort to assisted reproductive technologies, such as in vitro fertilization. Unfortunately, the lack of knowledge about a disease does not prohibit one from passing it on to somebody else. If you have sex with someone who is carrying a sexually transmitted disease, you can get it, too.

Remember, your eyes won't keep you sexually safe, your *mind* will.

STDs can be spread through vaginal, oral, and anal sex. Some can also be spread through any contact between the penis, vagina, mouth, or anus, even without intercourse. Sexually transmitted diseases can be spread from man to woman, woman to man, man to man, and woman to woman. Several STDs can be spread from mother to child at birth or through breast milk. And, as you probably are already aware, sharing needles can spread STDs, such as HIV.

There is only one way to be 100 percent sure you don't get a sexually transmitted disease: to remain abstinent. But for those of us interested in becoming sexually masterful that does seem a trifle unrealistic, does it not? Almost equally as safe, which we'll get into thoroughly in Chapter 6, is to give and receive pleasure solely by the use of the hands. Provided your hands have no open wounds, abrasions, or cracked skin, this form of sexual pleasure is virtually risk free, and with a bit of know-how and creativity, manual stimulation can be a most fulfilling form of sexual pleasure. Still, variety is the spice of life, and even the most exciting form of pleasure in exclusion of all others can become monotonous after a while.

What we *can* do is make sex as safe as possible and dramatically reduce the risk of contracting an STD. Meeting a stranger's eyes across a crowded room and falling into bed with him without so much as an exchange of names is a scene best left for Fantasy Island. Responsible adults talk about sex beforehand. Until you've both tested negative for all sexually transmitted diseases and waited the appropriate incubation period to ensure a clean bill of health (without engaging in any risk behaviors, such as unprotected sex with another partner or IV drug use), you should agree up front to use condoms *every single time* you engage in vaginal, oral, or anal sex. Condoms are now available for men and women, so you should *both* carry some at all times just in case. Even genital-to-genital contact without intercourse can transmit STDs such as HIV or syphilis. Foreplay involving any contact at all without condoms can be a problem.

Now, the female condom will protect you from unwanted pregnancy, and from diseases obtained through vaginal and anal sex. But it will not protect you from diseases that can be contracted by oral sex, as regular condoms can.

You can also reduce the risk of contracting an STD by limiting your sexual partners. You are more likely to get a sexually transmitted disease if *either* of you has more than one partner. That's why the value of trust should never go underestimated in a relationship. What is often brushed aside or chalked up as one little indiscretion could literally be a matter of life and death. This is not a judgment; it's a fact. If you can justify a reason to cheat on your lover or spouse, that's your business. But please, be safe.

Finally, if you use intravenous drugs, don't share needles.

The Diseases

The following is a list of common sexually transmitted diseases along with their symptoms, potential dangers, treatments, and cures. This list is for your general information. It is not wise, under any circumstances, to self-diagnose when it comes to personal health. Several of these symptoms can be caused by factors other than an STD, and as I said earlier, many STDs can exist for a very long time before *any* symptoms are noticeable. If you think you have an STD, see your doctor. Smarter still, if you have engaged in risk behaviors, for your (and your partner's) health, get tested during a regular physical exam.

If your physician confirms your suspicions, follow the medication instructions to the letter, and tell you partner or partners immediately. There is no question that this can be difficult to do. But if your partner is not treated, too, he or she can easily give the disease back to you or to someone else, as well as be at risk of having irreparable damage. For more information about these and other sexually transmitted diseases, you can call the National STD Hotline at (800) 227–8922.

CHLAMYDIA is often called the silent STD because there are usually no symptoms until the disease is in an advanced state. Symptoms may include burning during urination, unusual discharge from your vagina, pain in the lower abdomen, pain during sex, and bleeding between periods. An estimated four million new cases will be contracted by women in the U.S. this year alone. Chlamydia is spread through oral sex and intercourse. It can cause a bacterial infection deep within the fallopian tubes, causing chronic pain, tubal pregnancies, and infertility. With oral transmission, chlamydia will give you an upper respiratory infection. Chlamydia can be passed from mother to child during birth, causing eye and lung infections in newborns. The good news is that chlamydia is easily cured with antibiotics, but it must be tested for specifically. This test is not included in a regular Pap smear. You have to ask your doctor to be tested for it. Symptoms for men are pain during urination and discharge from the penis.

GONORRHEA, also referred to as "the clap," is similar to chlamydia, in that it is a bacterial infection that often goes undetected in women until permanent damage has already occurred. While we tend to associate gonorrhea with another century, the disease is still rampant in our country today. Although the number of cases of gonorrhea has dropped dramatically, it is still a common infection in adolescents. If left untreated, it can cause sterility, tubal pregnancies, and chronic pain. It can also lead to pelvic inflammatory disease (PID). Gonorrhea can be passed from mother to child during birth, causing eye, ear, and lung infections. Symptoms can include a yellow pus-like discharge from the vagina, pain while urinating, the need to urinate often, pain in the lower abdomen, and bleeding between periods. However, gonorrhea can also be completely asymptomatic. The good news is that this disease is easily curable if detected early with antibiotics. This STD is *highly* contagious and can be spread through any contact with the penis, vagina, mouth, or anus even without penetration. Men's symptoms are discharge from the penis and pain during urination.

Here's an interesting story related to me by a forty-two-year-old business executive for a Fortune 500 company, who had just come out of an eleven-month relationship when she had her annual OB-GYN appointment. She told her doctor that she thought she might have a yeast infection. The doctor told her that, as a matter of course, she would run a series of tests on her that checked for *all* STDs. What strikes me about this example is how quick the doctor was to check for STDs: that's how ubiquitous they are. She did just have a yeast infection but was also glad to know she was "clean."

PELVIC INFLAMMATORY DISEASE (PID) is most often the result of advanced stages of chlamydia or gonorrhea. It is the leading cause of infertility in the United States. The most common symptom of PID is pain in the lower abdomen. Other symptoms include bleeding between periods, increased amount of, or a change in, vaginal discharge, nausea or vomiting, and fever with chills. When detected early, PID is not life threatening, but if there has been damage to the fallopian tubes before detection, the consequences are often permanent.

SYPHILIS is a very dangerous bacterial infection. It is very rare today in the general population. If left untreated, syphilis can be fatal or cause irreparable damage to the heart, brain, eyes, and joints. Forty percent of all babies born to mothers with syphilis die during childbirth. They can also be born with abnormal features. Symptoms are painless sores, rashes on the palms and feet, and swollen lymph nodes. If the ulcer or rash is present, syphilis is highly contagious through oral, vaginal, and anal sex, as well as through open wounds on the skin. When detected early, syphilis is curable with strong doses of antibiotics. Men's symptoms are the same as for women.

TRICHOMONIASIS (TRICH) is a form of vaginitis caused by an amoeba-like organism that is spread through intercourse. An estimated three million new cases of vaginitis will be contracted in the U.S. this year. Not all forms of vaginitis are sexually transmitted, but the symptoms are similar. Yeast infections are a very common form of vaginitis not necessarily spread through sexual contact. You can get vaginitis by douching, taking antibiotics, adhering to a poor diet, and using vaginal products such as lubricants, sprays, and birth control devices. In addition, scented soaps, deodorants, detergents, and dyes in underwear or toilet tissue can also cause it. Symptoms can include discharge that is white or gray with an unusual odor, itching in or around the vagina, pain during sex, and pain during urination. It is more uncomfortable than harmful. Vaginitis is easily treatable through a prescription medication and by some medications sold over the counter.

HERPES is another common STD. What's most startling about genital herpes is how widespread it is among the American population. It is estimated that somewhere between 200,000 and 500,000 new cases of genital herpes will be contracted this year and 30 million Americans are infected already. An accountant from Milwaukee was shocked with how she had contracted the virus. She told me that after having been celibate for more than three years, she had slept with a man she worked with. She and he were friends, and after a few drinks after work one Friday, they went back to her place and ended up in bed together. Not more than three weeks later, she noticed she had painful, open sores on her labia. She went to the doctor, who confirmed that she had herpes. Then she called her friend. He was shocked: since he had never experienced an outbreak, he was completely unaware that he carried the herpes virus.

There are two types of herpes virus: the herpes simplex virus 1 (HSV I) and 2 (HSV II). HSV 2 causes genital herpes more often, but the HSV types 1 and 2 DNA can cause both genital herpes and cold sores. Visible symptoms include painful and/or itchy bumps or blisters near or inside the vagina and/or the rectum on women, and on the genital area for men, typically near the head of the penis. The virus can be contracted through any mucous membrane, including the eyes or any break in the skin. The first outbreak of genital herpes usually lasts between twelve and fourteen days, while subsequent outbreaks are shorter in duration (four to five days) and milder. Herpes is highly contagious when physical contact is made during an outbreak, but, as demonstrated by my seminar attendee's case, it can also be contagious when the virus lies dormant. There is no cure for this virus, though the oral medications Acyclovir, Valcyclorir, and Famcyclorir have proven to be highly successful in both minimizing the symptoms of current outbreaks and suppressing future recurrences.

What, precisely, causes a herpes recurrence has not been determined. However, studies indicate there is a strong association between herpes outbreaks and stress. While the symptoms of herpes can be very uncomfortable to those who have it, the real danger of this sexually transmitted disease is to an unborn child or an autoimmune-suppressed individual—someone with HIV or AIDS, for example. Most often transmitted during delivery, herpes can cause painful blisters and damage to the eyes, brain, and internal organs of a newborn baby. One in six newborns with herpes will not survive at all. The good news is that when knowledge of the herpes virus exists, a cesarean delivery can prevent damage to the child.

HPV (HUMAN PAPILLOMA VIRUS INFECTION), also known as condyloma, is a family of viruses consisting of over seventy different types. It is probably the most common STD. There will be an estimated one million new cases of HPV diagnosed this year. Certain forms of HPV cause visible genital warts, though some strains of HPV infection cause no warts at all. Genital warts are growths that appear on the vulva, in or around the vagina or anus, and on the cervix, penis, scrotum, groin, or thigh. They can be raised or flat, single or multiple, small or large. All sexually active men and women are susceptible to contracting HPV. It is spread by direct contact during vaginal, oral, and anal sex with someone who has the virus.

There is often confusion about HPV and its relation to cervical cancer. There are two types of HPV that are known to cause cervical cancer and several others that specifically cause genital warts but not cervical cancer. Because is it is a virus that can lie dormant for years, there is no known cure for this disease. Genital warts can be treated in several ways including freezing, laser surgery, chemical peels, and topical creams. The strains of HPV that don't produce genital warts usually go undetected until there is an abnormality in your Pap smear. The good news is that genital HPV is manageable with proper diagnosis and cervical cancer has a high rate of cure when detected in its earliest stages. For this reason, it is imperative for all women to have regular gynecological checkups. Research suggests that about 30 percent of people who have had sex carry HPV. This rate is even higher in certain age groups and locales. For men, the painless growths that usually appear on the penis may also appear on the urethra or in the rectal area.

HEPATITIS B is a disease of the liver. At least two causes of hepatitis can be sexually transmitted, hepatitis B virus (HBV) and hepatitis C (HCV). These infections are not curable and are much more infectious than HIV. It is spread through infected semen, vaginal secretions, and saliva, and it is easily passed from mother to unborn child. You can get Hepatitis B from vaginal, oral, and anal sex. You can also get it by direct contact with an infected person through open sores and cuts. If someone in your home is infected, you can contract Hepatitis B by using the same razor or toothbrush. You can even get this disease by wearing the same pierced earrings as someone who has it. In its mildest and most common form, you may never know you have it, but a few carriers develop cirrhosis and/or liver cancer. Your chances of contracting liver cancer are two hundred times higher if you've had these viral infections. Symptoms, when they appear, can be very much like those of the stomach flu. See your doctor immediately if you have nausea, unexplainable tiredness, dark urine, or yellowing of the eyes and skin. The treatment for the disease is rest and a diet high in both protein and carbohydrates. There is a vaccination for Hepatitis B, consisting of a series of shots, given in the arm. You must have all three shots to be safe. Hepatitis B mainly attacks young men and women in their teens and twenties, but once you contract it, you're a carrier for life. This year in the U.S., there will be more than 300,000 new cases of Hepatitis B documented. Not all doctors and nurses are aware of this fast-growing problem in their communities, so don't be afraid to ask for your vaccination.

HIV/AIDS—
The Epidemic Does Continue

ACQUIRED IMMUNODEFICIENCY SYNDROME (AIDS) is caused by human immunodeficiency virus (HIV) infection. When someone tests positive for HIV, it means his or her system has been exposed to HIV and has produced an immune response. HIV and AIDS are not the same thing; one is the precursor of the other. You cannot get AIDS without having the HIV infection. You can, however, test positive for the HIV infection without having an AIDS diagnosis.

An AIDS diagnosis occurs when you have:

i) A postive HIV test and an AIDS defining opportunistic infection. There are approximately twenty-five known opportunistic infections.

ii) A positive HIV test and a T-cell count under 200 per cubic millimeter of blood.

iii) A positive HIV test and pulmonary tuberculosis, invasive cervical cancer, or recurrent bacterial pneumonia.

HIV attacks the immune system, leaving the body unable to fight off common sicknesses or other diseases. Somewhere between 600,000 to 900,000 people in the U.S. are infected with HIV.

HIV infection can be spread through blood, semen and vaginal fluids, and to infants through breast milk. Touching, eating, coughing, mosquitoes, toilet seats, swimming in pools, and donating blood do NOT spread HIV. What is rare but can occur is transmission from kissing a highly infected person; it is more likely that when HIV is contracted through kissing, the transmission occurs through blood than through saliva, resulting from extremely poor oral hygiene (in other words, through open sores in the mouth). HIV is not an airborne virus and cannot be spread by casual contact.

There are usually no symptoms accompanying HIV. People can get the virus and feel terrific for many years. Unfortunately, the virus almost always leads to AIDS eventually, and because it is the immune system that fails, the symptoms for AIDS can look like anything from a cold to cancer. Although there is no cure for AIDS, there are new drugs that dramatically slow down the effect that HIV has on the immune system. Every sexually active man and woman should have an HIV test and wait the six months required to ensure a clean bill of health before having sex without a male condom.

Sadly, it isn't always enough to accept a verbal declaration of good health. Many, many people have been deceived by lovers who claimed to be HIV-negative and weren't. Sharon, the girl-friend of a seminar attendee, had a whirlwind romance with a sports newscaster and married him in a romantic ceremony on the fifty-yard-line of his alma mater. Shortly after returning from their honeymoon, she was disturbed by his sudden lack of inter-est in sex. After a few months, the marriage quickly deteriorated and they were divorced within a year, but not before Sharon discovered she was pregnant. Although her ex-husband seemed excited about becoming a father, his initial enthusiasm gave way to less and less frequent visits with his young daughter. Then, one day while Sharon was watching Dan Rather do an interview with a man dying of AIDS her heart sank. Although the man's face was shielded from the camera and his voice was altered, because of his mannerisms and the fact that he was wearing a sweater she had given him on a past Christmas, Sharon realized that this dying man was indeed her ex-husband and the father of her daughter. The next day she went to get tested and discovered that she was HIV-positive.

It is very important that you ask to see the results of your lover's HIV test and all his tests for sexually transmitted diseases, especially if you don't know him well, but even if you do. It is also important that he see the results of your tests. Rather than make him ask, it is a good idea if you offer the results as a show of good faith, opening the door for him to do the same. If your lover refuses to show you his test results, *you* refuse to have unprotected sex with him. Remember, it is your health and quite possibly your life, that is affected by his being secretive. No one would want to keep his or her *good* health a secret.

When obtaining an HIV test, be mindful of the difference between *confidential* and *anonymous* testing. They are not the same. When you have an anonymous test, you are identified by a number or letters only, not by your name, your social security number, or any other identifying information. After the blood sample is taken, you confirm that the numbers and letters on the vial and on your identification slip are the same. A week later you go back to the clinic where the test was taken and get the results. No results are given over the phone.

A confidential test means that the results are confidential, but the confidentiality is limited by the integrity of those who have access to the information. Sadly, only last year, an employee at a southern clinic ran off a list with the names of all those who had tested positive for HIV and sold it at a local bar—so much for confidential testing.

I'd like to make several important points about HIV/AIDS:

1. There are several strains of the HIV virus. So even if a man or a woman is already positive, he or she can still become infected by another form of the virus and in fact is even more susceptible, given the already weakened state of the immune system.

2. HIV-positive means you have been exposed to the HIV virus, which causes AIDS. Your body shows a positive immune response to the HIV virus. In 1993, the CDC established a definition benchmark for the diagnosis of AIDS, enabling physicians to differentiate between testing positive for HIV and AIDS. This set parameters for qualifying people for health insurance coverage and research programs.

3. Some strains are nastier than others. Depending on the virulence of the strain one is exposed to, you could develop AIDS almost immediately.

4. It is suggested that you wait six months after risk behavior before getting tested, because it can take up to six months for antibodies to show up in a test. Most people (95 percent) test positive within three months of exposure.

5. In 1998, the CDC estimates that 50 percent of people who are HIV-positive do not know they are infected.

6. An opportunistic infection is a life threatening infection that in a healthy normal immune system would not be threatening, but for someone with a compromised immune system the infection takes the "opportunity" to attack the already weakened system. For example, a person who is undergoing cancer treatment such as chemotherapy is at risk for an opportunistic infection. Opportunistic infections are *not* all possible infections; they are caused by a limited number of fungi, protozoa, bacteria, and viruses.

Condom Mania

While I've discussed the most common of the sexually transmitted diseases, there are more than fifty known STDs to date. By providing you with knowledge about them I don't mean to scare you, but rather to empower you. No one should have to be frightened into taking control of his or her sexual health. Rather, now that you have this information, I hope being safe and careful becomes a matter of self-respect for you. There just isn't an excuse good enough to not practice safe sex in a relationship with someone whose health you're not 100 percent sure about.

You don't drive without car insurance. You don't go through life without health or home insurance. Latex condoms are the best possible sex insurance available. When it comes to protecting yourself from pregnancy you can get away with forgetting your birth control many times without getting caught. But it only takes *one* encounter without protection to contract a sexually transmitted disease. Is it worth risking your life?

CHOOSING A CONDOM

There are many different condoms to choose from, but not all of them are of the same quality.

Condom Tips to Remember

- Although you may hear differently, spermicides containing Nonoxynol-9 were created to help reduce the risk of unwanted pregnancy, *not* sexually transmitted diseases. Spermicides should be used only in *addition* to condoms, never in place of them. Nonoxynol-9 is a detergent-like substance that has proven to be effective at killing HIV in *laboratory* tests ONLY. There is nothing conclusive at this time to indicate Nonoxynol-9 kills HIV in human beings. I have, however, been told by many women that they have traced their chronic vaginal and/or bladder infections back to this highly irritating substance found in some creams, gels, lubricants, and on condoms.

- Avoid buying condoms manufactured in China or Korea, where poor quality latex is often used.

- Beware of condoms labeled as "novelty" (e.g., "glow-in-the-dark" condom). These are not intended to provide pregnancy or STD protection.

Type of condom	Lubricated/ non-lubric	Available with/ without spermicide	Type of lubricant to use
LATEX			
Kimono- microthin	lubricated	both	water based
Lifestyles Xtra Pleasure	lubricated	both	water based
Crown Skin Less Skin	lubricated	both	water based
Vis-à-vis Ultrathin	lubricated	both	water based
Magnum	lubricated	both	water based
Trojan Ultra Pleasure	lubricated	both	water based
Class Act Ultra Thin and Sensitive	lubricated	both	water based
Lifestyles Ultra Thin	lubricated	both	water based
Contempo Wet 'n' Wild	lubricated	both	water based
NATURAL			
Fourex Skins *or* Naturalamb Skin Kling Tite	lubricated	both	water based— if needed
POLYURETHENE			
Reality for Women	lubricated	without	water or oil based
Avanti for Men	lubricated	Available only with spermicide	water or oil based

Variations: 1: *Colored* 2: *Textured* 3: *Scented* 4: *Slim fit* 5: *Size*	Cost	Where to purchase: -*drugstore* -*supermarket* -*mail order* -*convenience stores* -*Internet*	Field researcher comments
None	Average	D/S/M/C/I	Light, strong
5: Designed with an oversized end that heightens sensation and friction during thrusting	Average	D/S/M/C/I	New product bringing back great idea
none	Average	D/S/M/C/I	It's so sheer, nice pinky color
none	Average	D/S/M/C/I	Felt great
5: Best of the large size condoms	Average	D/S/M/C/I	Best for Italian Method (see p.76)
none	Average	D/S/M/C/I	Know the name–great new product, nice and thin
none	Average	D/S/M/C/I	Light
2: studded, ribbed 3: Kiss of Mint	Average	D/S/M/C/I	Easy to get, felt good
1: Midnight 4: Snug fit	Average	D/S/M/C/I	Loved the box, we liked the thinness
none	Expensive	D/S/M/C/I	Great protection against pregnancy when not concerned with STDs
none	Expensive	Best thru mail order or Internet if difficult to find retail	All-around great protection for women
none	Average to Expensive	D/S/M/C/I	Too much breakage

- If you're shy about purchasing condoms, there are several mail order catalogues available. See the Sources section at the end of the book.

- There is a male polyurethane condom on the market, Avanti, which states on its own box that:

  "The risks of pregnancy and sexually transmitted diseases (STDs), including AIDS (HIV infection), are not known for this condom. A study is being done."

  So, in combination with the high rate of breakage that our field researchers experienced with this condom—over 25 percent—I cannot in good conscience recommend this product until their "study" is done.

- The FEMALE polyurethane condom called REALITY is made by a different manufacturer; it is thicker, stronger, and overall an outstanding product. It is possible to insert the REALITY condom hours before one is intimate and one can also use an oil- or water-based lubricant. It is ideal for those who are latex sensitive and has the added bonus of being adaptable for anal sex. However, while the need for female-controlled barrier methods is great, the performance of this condom leaves a lot to be desired. The pregnancy rates are 12 percent for six months, meaning twenty-four pregnancies per year if one hundred women rely on this condom.

- The most popular line of condoms ordered by the legal prostitution "ranches," or "establishments," of Nevada are Ansell condoms: Prime, Contempo, and Lifestyles—without Nonoxynol-9.

CONDOMS BREAK

Any condom can break during intercourse, and for many different reasons. Keep in mind these considerations when using condoms:

- Breakage is invariably a result of improper handling such as using your teeth to open the foil, keeping condoms in wallets for extended periods of time, or using a lubricant with an oil base.

- During a study conducted by Dr. Bruce Voeller, founder of the Mariposa Foundation, men who were chronic condom breakers were discovered to have been using everyday hand lotion as a lubricant. A lubricant must be water-based and most hand lotions contain some form of oil. Oil is a latex condom's mortal enemy because it immediately begins to break down the latex. Therefore it is imperative that the ingredients of a lotion be checked carefully before using it with a latex condom. Better still, use a lubricant *intended* for this use, such as Astroglide, Sensura, or K-Y, rather than letting him grab the closest bottle of lotion off your vanity. It *must* be water-based. (There is more complete information on lubrication in the next chapter.)

- The most common excuse I hear from women who have had unprotected sex is that their lovers don't like condoms because they diminish the male pleasure factor. I won't lie to you; men attest to the truth of this lessening of pleasure. However, after you both have waited the six-month period to make sure you're both healthy, you will be free and clear to use other methods of birth control. He may have to endure a slightly diminished sensation while you're using condoms, but remember that you can always give him a hand job without risk, providing your hands have no abrasions or open wounds.

- One of the excuses I hear from men in my seminars is that they are too big to fit into any of the condoms currently available. Whenever I hear a man saying this I know a simple yet most effective response: simply open a regular size condom, shape your fingers into a bird's beak, and, watching your nails, unroll the condom over your hand. Pull it down, stretching it so that it covers your entire forearm past your elbow (it *will* fit, trust me). Then ask him how much bigger than that he is. Whenever I do this in the ladies' seminar, there is a great deal of laughter.

- Some men are likely to be more comfortable in a bigger condom. If your lover has a thick, broad penis, a regular size condom may fit a little too snugly at the base of his shaft or at the head. There is no reason for him to suffer. For this reason condoms also come in larger sizes.

The Italian Method

There is a way I've found that rarely fails to make a man welcome the application of a condom. I have dubbed it "The Italian Method," but it is actually an old trick that has been used by "working girls" since the invention of the condom. This isn't a reinvention of any wheel, but the renaming of a much-used wheel. The name is strictly a marketing term and has nothing to do with Italian men, an old Italian boyfriend, or anything at all Italian. I simply needed a code name that was acceptable to polite society.

Simply put, The Italian Method is the application of a condom using your mouth, and men absolutely go crazy for it. A thirty-eight-year-old female computer executive from Dallas put it this way: "I used to hate having to put on a condom. It always seemed to put a damper on the mood. When I perform The Italian Method, the mood is anything but dampened! In fact, it puts me *more* in the mood to make love."

Secret from Lou's Archives

If his pubic hair is too thick for you, you might want to consider trimming it. You can even make it part of your foreplay.

A few years ago a woman came to me who was very unsure about the prospect of having good safe sex with her new boyfriend. This woman was fifty-two at the time and a fashion designer. Although she and her lover had thoroughly discussed and agreed to be responsible about their sexual relationship, she was recently divorced and was completely unfamiliar with the condom "etiquette" of the nineties. She had many questions including, but not limited to, who was supposed to bring the condom. We ended up talking for hours on the subject, during which time I showed her how to perform The Italian Method. When she finally left to meet her lover for their first tryst, the woman was brimming with confidence, not only in her ability to artfully apply a condom in this manner, but also in the fact that being sexually responsible carries its own heat.

Upon arriving for their first intimate encounter, he pulled out a condom (though her overnight bag contained a supply as well) and sheepishly asked, "Do you know how to put this thing on?"

The woman looked at him and answered honestly, "Only with my mouth."

He couldn't believe his ears and asked her to repeat her response. Again she said, "Only with my mouth." When he questioned how on earth she knew how to do this, the woman explained to him she had taken a class on sexual technique and safety. The reason, she told him, was because she didn't want to compromise the fun and sensuality of their intimate relationship for the responsible approach they had agreed to take in ensuring that their sex was as risk free as possible. He was overwhelmed by both her mastery of The Italian Method and the effort she had taken to make their intimate relationship so special. Although they've been together now for nearly four years, he still says it was what he learned about her character on that day that made him fall deeply in love.

As much as I enjoy relating this story, I want to reiterate that I spent a great deal of one-on-one time with this woman, giving her plenty of opportunity to make mistakes in the beginning. The Italian Method *does* take a bit of practice (I suggest using either a dildo or a cucumber). But you must trust me on this: the effect it has on your lover will be eternal. As a male screenwriter from Los Angles remarked, "The whole thing is hot! I love watching her breasts as she goes down on me and feeling the heat and pressure of her mouth as she makes her way down my shaft. I feel like we're the stars of our own erotic film."

Before you begin, please take note that only latex condoms are to be used for The Italian Method. "Natural" material condoms not only taste terrible, their only protective value is in the prevention of pregnancy. Natural material condoms are made from animal membranes and this tissue will stop the much larger sperm but not the tiny STD virus particles that could infect you.

Secret from Lou's Archives

Ladies, when using The Italian Method, please remove any lipstick or lip gloss, as its oils will break down a latex condom and make it ineffective as protection.

But first, in order to proceed, you need to be able to do two things: 1) put your mouth in a flute position (like a baby kissing), and 2) cover your teeth with your lips and open your mouth.

HOW TO PERFORM
THE ITALIAN METHOD
*There are six steps involved in The Italian Method,
none of which can be forgotten or discarded:*

Step 1. Lube your lips with a clear, water-based lubricant (while a colored lubricant won't harm you, it may leave you looking like Bozo the Clown). You can either apply the lube to your lips yourself or have him do it for you.

Step 2. A package of three condoms should be plenty. Don't buy a slew—guys will make assumptions. Then, remove a condom from its package and place it in position to be unrolled. If you hold the nipple between your thumb and forefinger and it

4

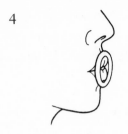

resembles the shape of a sombrero hat, held by its top, it is in the right position to be unrolled correctly. If the edges of the sombrero are flipped under, you will not be able to unroll it down the shaft.

5

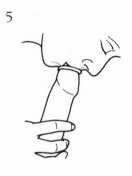

Step 3. Once you have the condom in the correct position, invert it so that it looks like a mini upside-down sombrero. Place a dollop* of water-based lubricant *only* in the receptacle (nipple) end of the latex condom, as if you were putting it in the finger of a latex glove. The lubricant here has two functions: it will allow the condom to slip gently over the most sensitive part of his penis (the head), preventing that stuck-to-the-top feeling men complain about so often. In addition, it will give the condom more range of motion during sexual activity, which translates into more sensation for him.

6

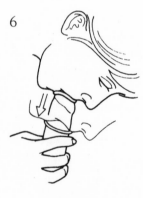

Note: Steps 4, 5, and 6 must be done quickly so that the lubricant doesn't run out over the shaft of the penis.

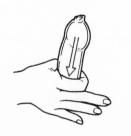

* A dollop, in this case, should be approximately the size of a regular jelly bean. If you use more than that amount here, you could end up lubing his shaft, which could result in the condom slipping off at an inopportune moment.

Step 4. Position your lips as if you were going to give someone a kiss, but with your lips not touching. You'll sort of resemble a choirboy for a minute, but that look is a fleeting one. Put the condom in your mouth, lubricated side toward him, and use a little suction to hold it in place. The rim of the sombrero will be outside your puckered lips, not inside.

Step 5. Hold the shaft of his penis in one hand and move your mouth to the top of the head of his penis. If you move too slowly, all the lubricant will drip out. Releasing the suction only slightly, allow the condom to rest on the head of the penis while you push it down gently with your tongue, removing any air bubbles.

Step 6. Staying in this position, quickly wrap your well-lubricated lips over your teeth and push gently but firmly in one smooth motion on the rim of the condom to unravel it down the shaft. The only way this will work is if your lips are wrapped firmly over your teeth. If they aren't, not only will you risk hurting him, you won't have the strength to push the condom down quickly. Your lips need the support of your teeth behind them in order for this technique to be effective. If you are unable to push the condom all the way down with your lips, don't worry about it. Very few woman can, at first. Go as far down as you are comfortable, finishing the job with your fingers in the shape of an "okay" sign to unroll the rest. Some women have said the sensation of coolness from the lube in the nipple end of the condom causes them to gag if they go down the shaft too far. If this should happen to you, you can complete the roll with your fingers in the shape of the "okay" sign.

Again, The Italian Method does take some practice, but it can be a lot of fun and very sensual once you get the hang of it.

If this is not something that appeals to you, however, don't feel pressured to make it part of your sexual repertoire, but keep in mind that there is no good excuse for not using a condom. Simply explain that until you *both* have assurance of your mutual good health, there is no sex without one. It's both practical and erotic: "I usually lose about 50 percent of my erection while fumbling to apply a condom. But when she did this, I didn't lose any of it at all! I couldn't believe it," said a stockbroker from Cleveland.

Secret from Lou's Archives

When choosing a latex condom for The Italian Method, avoid brands that are coated with Nonoxynol-9. It has a vile taste and will cause temporary numbing of your mouth.

In the next chapter, you will see how lubrication and its application can only increase the pleasure that is related to having fabulous sex without compromising your safety. Safety is essential, but it doesn't have to ruin the mood or lessen the charge between you and your lover. You should think of the information here as an expression of your respect for yourself, as well as your partner.

Chapter Five

To Lube or Not to Lube? There Is No Question

*"Who knew you could accomplish
so much with so little?"*

MALE SEMINAR ATTENDEE, AGE 32

The whole thing happened quite innocently. Early on in her marriage, a woman found she felt drier than she used to because of the birth control she was now using, a method known to cause dryness. After taking a quick shower, she decided to apply some lubricant to herself after her shower and before getting into bed with her husband. They began to kiss and, as will often happen, he slid his hand down to her genital area. Well, he was *so* proud and turned on by the obvious effect his kisses had on her she couldn't bear to tell him her wetness wasn't entirely his doing. Furthermore, he went on to make such mad passionate love to her that night that ten years into their marriage, she's *still* secretly applying lubricant to herself before many of their romantic encounters. He still thinks his kisses bring on Niagara Falls and she's still reaping the benefits.

While I'm not, as a rule, a proponent of one lover misleading another, in this particular case it *does* seem rather harmless, especially since she also keeps a bottle of personal lubricant by the bed at all times, which they use openly whenever they desire. For this reason and many others, I feel personal lubricant is quite simply a *treasure*. I can't think of a single store-bought item that does more to enhance the overall pleasure and ease of sexual technique than lubricant. That being so, I am constantly amazed at how many women have yet to discover the amount of joy that can be created from one little bottle. Those of you who have not tried it are in for a treat. As a thirty-nine-year-old male entrepreneur from Sacramento said, "I never knew her hand could feel so good."

Many women in my seminars have said they believe the use of personal lubricant is in some way a poor reflection on them. They tell me they are afraid that if they bring out a bottle of lubricant during lovemaking that their lovers may think they're incapable of getting excited "naturally." One woman put it suc-cinctly: "I don't use it every time, just sometimes to give me a physical jump start when I'm already there mentally." I've also had men tell me that they, too, are afraid to introduce lubricant during sex; from their point of view, they're afraid we women will think *they* aren't exciting enough to get *us* lubricated.

Secret from Lou's Archives
Women lubricate naturally, even while sleeping. Chances are, ladies, it has nothing to do with what he's doing to you.

Let me put both myths to rest: neither of those scenarios are correct. The fact that, as women, we have the ability to self-lubricate when we become sexually aroused is just another one of Mother Nature's many gifts. She didn't want us or our part-ners to be uncomfortable during intercourse. Of course, she didn't account for things like antibiotics, alcohol consumption, or a salty diet to interfere with her work, either. But they do. Mother Nature also didn't know we humans would find ways to make sexual encounters so intense that they'd go on for hours and involve far more than intercourse. Nor did she realize we'd find it thrilling to make love on the spur of the moment once in a while *without* taking the time for her gift to kick in. So we invented lubricant not to replace her gift, but rather to embellish it. After all, no two women are going to self-lubricate in the same amount or for the same reasons. What turns us on and how much we are affected changes constantly. And believe me, if you use lubricant, men will thank you. As one forty-two-year-old businessman from New York said, "I'm going to invent a tool belt, strap it on, with lubricant in one pocket, and a vibrator in the other."

The Right Lube for You

Beyond the biological reasons for using personal lubricant, it also provides an undeniable element of fun. I have a client who enjoys the benefits of lube to the extent that all she has to do is call her husband on the phone at the office and snap open the top of the bottle next to the receiver (she uses Midnight Fire—see below). He is so aware of the sound and what it means, she knows he'll do everything in his power to find a way to come home as soon as he can. Now, they call it their "phone foreplay."

Before I get into the fun of lube and its application, I want to help you figure out how to pick the right lubricant for your needs. If you've ever been in an adult novelty shop, you know there are MANY of them to choose from—water-based, oil-based, flavored, unflavored, scented, unscented, colored, clear, liquid, and gels. It can be a bit overwhelming.

There are a few details you should keep in mind when choosing a personal lubricant:

- Remember, oil and latex don't mix. Oil breaks down the latex in the condoms, often causing them to break. An oil-based lubricant is fine for manual sex, but if you're planning to continue on to intercourse using a condom, be sure to use a lubricant that is water-based. And when you're using water-based lubricants, if you find your lube is getting a little sticky or thick due to evaporation, a couple of additional drops of H_2O will return it to its full lubricity. There's more than one reason to keep a glass of water next to the bed.

- *Always* read the label of a lubricant in its entirety. The big print alone can be misleading sometimes. If you see the word "oil" listed anywhere under ingredients, chances are the product is not water based. If you are sensitive or susceptible to irritation, watch out for the spermicide known as Nonoxynol-9. It can be extremely irritating to both men and women. This is the active ingredient in contraceptive foam and jelly, suppositories, and contraceptive film. With the latter, you insert vaginally, and the heat and moisture "melt" the film to a consistency similar to jelly.

- Know what you're putting onto your body. Eros is a new silicone lubricant that describes itself as a "bodyglide." Eros, Millennium, and Platinum are three newer products that are made with dimethicone (silicone) and carry no protective value; they aren't water soluble. Fine for external use; I would be careful about internal.

FAVORITE LUBRICANTS FOR MANUAL SEX

I put together a team of field researchers to go and investigate which lubricants felt and tasted the best for different sexual activities. The results of our efforts are listed below, though this is by no means an exhaustive study. An asterisk denotes that the product is colorless.

- ASTROGLIDE.* The Astroglide company uses Second Only to Mother Nature as its byline, and our field researchers would have to agree this product is the closest to our own natural intimate moisture. Astroglide is one of the most popular and easy-to-find brands of water-based personal lubricant. It has a slightly sweet taste and is odorless. You can buy it at your local drugstore and in many supermarkets as well.

Secret from Lou's Archives

Many women I know prefer colorless lubricants, as they won't stain the sheets or any other material.

- SENSURA/SEX GREASE.* This is the water-based lubricant of choice for many connoisseurs. It is a clear thick liquid with a velvety texture that maintains its slick feel for a long time. The same product is market-

ed and packaged under two different names—for the
ladies it is called Sensura and bottled in pink, for the
men it is called Sex Grease and bottled in black.

- K-Y LIQUID.* This is the water-based liquid version
  of the classic lube. It is very similar to Astroglide in
  texture and taste.

- DELUBE.* This water-based lubricant is fairly new on
  the market. It has a nice light texture, and is tasteless
  and clear. Besides being a great all-around lubricating
  product, one of the best things about DeLube is its
  ability to heighten the skin's sensations. Benzalonium
  chloride (the active ingredient that causes the sensation) is used as a natural spermicide in Canada and
  throughout Europe.

- BODY WISE LIQUID SILK.* A water-based
  non-glycerine British product. Its creamy texture
  doesn't get sticky because there is no glycerine.

- MIDNITE FIRE.* This is the product that "snaps
  open." Midnite Fire will surely bring you lots of
  enjoyment. It not only comes in a variety of flavors, it
  also becomes very warm with gentle rubbing and even
  warmer when you blow on it following the rub. Not to
  worry, though—the heat only builds to a certain level
  so there is no risk of getting burned. Midnite Fire is a
  water-based lubricant that is safe for application both
  internally and externally. Although it is billed as The
  Hot Sensual Massage Lotion, it's really too thick to be
  used for a straight massage without adding water or
  another clear water-based lubricant. It feels especially
  erotic when applied to the nipples, inner thighs, the
  head of the penis, and the testicles.

- THE BODY SHOP PEPPERMINT FOOT LOTION.
  This one was a pleasant surprise, discovered by one of our more creative researchers. The mint allows for a cool feeling in combination with a tingly warmth created by repeated stroking. This *is* an oil-based product, however, which must be washed off completely before applying a latex condom. This one may also stain the sheets because it has oil in it. Start sparingly as too much may make him momentarily numb.

FAVORITE LUBRICANTS FOR ORAL SEX

At the risk of being annoying, I must again warn you to avoid, at all costs, using any lubricant containing the spermicidal Nonoxynol-9 during oral sex. This ingredient not only tastes awful, it will have a slight numbing effect on your mouth.

- ASTROGLIDE. Once again, Astroglide leads the pack because of its natural feel (light, odorless, tasteless) and how easy it makes it to do the techniques.

- SENSURA/SEX GREASE. Much like Astroglide, this is a favorite because of how it eases friction and heightens the manipulations while maintaining a natural feel. Some women say they detect a slight chemical taste in this product, but others don't taste anything at all.

- K-Y LIQUID. Field researchers rated this the same as Astroglide. Similar in taste and texture.

- MIDNITE FIRE. For those who like the sensation of taste during oral sex, Midnite Fire is a favorite because it comes in six different mouthwatering flavors— Cinnamon, Irish Cream, Strawberry, Cherry, Piña Colada, and Passion Fruit. Unlike other tested brands of lubricant, these flavors are not *so* sweet as to leave you nauseated.

- CHOCOLATE IN A JAR—LikkIt and LuvIt. Technically, this isn't a lube at all, but nonetheless, the researchers who liked it were absolutely crazy about this product so I thought it should be included. This is premium quality Belgian chocolate in six luscious flavors: chocolate almond, chocolate extreme, white chocolate, chocolate supreme, chocolate raspberry, and chocolate mocha. Spread this delicately over each others' bodies and lick it off. The only downside to this product is that it needs to be refrigerated between uses, which requires a few seconds in the microwave before lubricating with it so it isn't too cold. Still, the taste and texture are divine.

It is not for the calorie-conscious, however, nor is it to be used with latex condoms because of the butterfat (an oil) contained in the chocolate.

FAVORITE LUBRICANTS FOR INTERCOURSE

- SENSURA/SEX GREASE. This one beat out Astroglide for use during intercourse because of its slightly thicker, velvety texture. All the researchers agreed that there is something heavenly about making love with the help of Sensura/Sex Grease.

- ASTROGLIDE. What can I say? For anyone who wants the benefit of extra comfort during intercourse, but doesn't want to feel anything even the slightest bit unnatural, Astroglide is the lubricant of choice.

FAVORITE LUBRICANTS FOR SEX TOYS

When applying lubricant for the purpose of comfort when using sex toys, I recommend sticking to those that are water based, clear, and fragrance-free. Some of the newer plastic and silicone compounds of which the toys are made tend to break down over time when exposed to oil. And anytime you use a product that has dye or fragrance in it, you run the risk (even if only a slight one) of having an allergic reaction when you use it internally. Most companies (certainly the ones mentioned above) go to great lengths to test their ingredients for potential allergic reactions. But no one can guarantee it won't ever happen to someone who is especially sensitive in those extremely delicate areas of the human body. I believe it is always better to be safe than sorry.

The Fun of Lubrication: Application

As one of my male clients said to me, "The best thing I learned about lubricants: I didn't know they could be so much fun!" Once you've chosen the right lube for your personal needs and desires, it is time for the fun to begin! So often this great opportunity to heighten the pleasure and overall erotic atmosphere of the sensual experience is overshadowed by a pedestrian method of lubricant application: just blopping it on.

Ladies, as we've already discussed, men tend to be very visual creatures. Why not take advantage of it? There are *much* better ways to go about applying lubricant and I'm going to share with you some of them right now.

Secret from Lou's Archives

Whether you're pouring into your hand, his hand, or somewhere else, try pouring the lubricant from a distance of at least 6 inches to add to the visual for him and prowess for you. Just blobbing lubricant into your hand is pedestrian.

ONE-HAND APPLICATION TECHNIQUES

- No Dominance. Pour the lube into your nondominant hand (the one you don't write with) and apply it with that one. In the same way that a drawing you did with your nondominant hand would be more free and less structured, so it is with the way you apply the lubricant. You'll also get a different awareness about the feel and texture of his penis than you do when touching him with your dominant hand.

- Playing Elsewhere. Pour a little pool of lubricant into *his* hand, bellybutton, or, if he's laying on his stomach, the small of his back and dip your fingers into the pool to apply the lube elsewhere. Because the skin is our largest organ, this will expand the sexual sensation to other areas of the body rather than limiting it to just the obvious hot spots.

TWO-HAND APPLICATION TECHNIQUES

- Together from the Top Down. Starting at the head of his penis, work your already lubricated hands down slowly, massaging his entire shaft and testicles in warm moisture.

- It Takes Two. He will be guiding your already lubricated hands as his applicators. Let him move them up and down his shaft, artfully applying the lubricant with the speed and pressure that feels best to him.

Secret from Lou's Archives

Have him pour some lubricant into your cupped hands. By then rubbing your hands together seductively, you'll not only warm up the lube, but you'll also let him know how good it feels to you and how good you are soon going to make *him* feel.

- Perfumery. Apply the lubricant to the inside of your forearms. Using the entire area between your wrists and your elbows, work his penis gently back and forth between them.

NO-HAND APPLICATION TECHNIQUES

- Self Improvement I & II (I is using one hand, II is using two hands). Ask your gentleman to give you either one or both of his hands. (Be sure to *ask*. Remember, the mainstay of all healthy sexual interaction is the culmination of permission requested followed by permission granted.) Once he has given you his hand(s), pour about a quarter-size dollop of Midnite Fire into the palm area. Using a couple of your fingers, spread the lube into his palm(s) as if you were painting them. Be sure to use enough motion to get the Midnite Fire warm. Ask him to let you know when he begins to feel the heat. When he does, lean toward his hands, and blow on his palm(s) to make them even warmer. The closer you are to the palm the more intense the heat. Finally, place your hands on the outside of his, this time using *his* hands as the applicator for the lubricant.

- The Dip. With him leaning or sitting up at a 45-degree angle and penis erect, pour a small stream of lubricant into his bellybutton. Gently push his penis toward his body, dipping the head into the pool you created and thus preparing him for whatever sexual activity you have in mind for him next.

- The Palm Reader (The Waterfall). From a distance of approximately twelve inches, pour a long, slow, generous stream of lubricant into the palm of your hand. Squeeze your fingers against your palm, allowing the lube to make a wonderful noise (men are not only visual creatures when it comes to sex, ladies, they are quite the auditory creatures, too). When the liquid has warmed sufficiently, turn your hand sideways and let the lubricant dribble out of the side of your clenched hand down over his soft, semierect, or erect penis. By the time all the liquid has spilled from your hand, his penis is much more likely to be the latter rather than the former. It's best to use Astroglide, as it is the most liquidy.

- The Madonna (The French F_____). Ask him to pour a generous amount of lubricant over your breasts. You can either rub it around for warmth yourself (men just *adore* watching women play with their own breasts) or have him do it for you (men also adore doing the playing themselves). Once your breasts are warm and thoroughly moistened, move your upper torso to his penis, using your breasts as the lube applicator.

LUBRICANT TIPS

- It's possible to use too much lubricant. Although it takes quite a bit to have too much, you'll both realize you've gone overboard with the lube when it causes the sensation to diminish. The good news is, it's easy to wipe away (particularly those that are water based). Keep a towel or tissues nearby.

- The best places to use lubricant are on and around the areas of insertion, toys, fingers, or any other thing which is to be inserted, and any areas that will be rubbed or stroked. After reading Chapters 6 and 7, you'll have a clearer idea not only about where to use lubricant, but about just how amazing this wonderful product really is.

- Try to avoid getting lubricant in your eyes. Oil-based lubricants can sting. The water-based variety generally won't sting, but they can temporarily blur your vision. Beyond that, where one does or does not enjoy the feeling of lubricant is a matter of personal preference. If you have a predisposition to bladder or vaginal infections, you should be very careful with *any* lubricant you are using. Some women are very sensitive to any fluid that affects their vagina's natural pH including, but not limited to, soaps and toilet tissues.

Whichever method of lubricant application you choose, be it one of these or one of your own creation, the most important advice I can share with you is to have *fun*. The application of the lube can add as much to the sensual experience as the function of the lube. Yet sometimes, using lube is bound to get messy. One of you might slip and pour too much, or the bottle could fall and you may just find yourselves sliding down the hallway. Don't worry. Lubricant is easy to clean up and easy to replace. The only thing of real value either of you is ever at risk of losing are your smiles.

Chapter Six

Give That Man a Hand

MASTERING
MANUAL STIMULATION

*"After attending the seminar and learning these techniques, I tried
them out immediately on returning home to my husband.
The only audible words I could decipher in his reaction
were, 'Oh Jesus, Mary, and Joseph.'
Funny thing—he's Jewish."*

FEMALE SEMINAR ATTENDEE,
MEDICAL DIRECTOR, AGE 28

Foreplay Is Mainplay

Sexually speaking, your life may be about to change forever.
Literally. Out of all the material I've collected through research,
personal experiences, and feedback through hundreds and hundreds of seminars, learning the techniques of manual stimulation seems to produce the most dramatic results in couples' intimate relations. And these techniques are typically what women
go home and try first after a seminar.

As you'll soon find out, a good hand job is an incredibly easy
skill to master (though *that* detail is best kept between us). Yet
the effect it has on a man is something he may lie awake and

dream about. And while I'm happy for the beneficiaries of this acquired skill, it's the effect it has on *women* that brings me the most satisfaction. One woman, a writer from Atlanta, described her experience this way:

> *I thought there was something wrong with me because I wasn't crazy about sex. I loved the* romance *part of it—the kissing, hugging, and snuggling—but the actual* mechanics *of sexual contact were always something for me to get through. Now I can see that I had mistaken my lack of knowledge for a lack of interest. Once I learned how to give the man I love this intense pleasure, our whole relationship changed. I am a willing participant in our sex life. It's really powerful. When I say powerful, I don't mean that I have power over* him *(although he insists that I do), I'm referring to a newfound closeness we have in every area. We are four years into our relationship, a time when many couples complain about a waning sense of lust. Our lust factor is at an all-time high and shows no signs of diminishing in the near future.*

Part of my point here is that sexual intercourse makes up a very small portion of the entire sexual experience. As I said earlier, intercourse is something for which we are biologically programmed, and it is merely the tip of the proverbial iceberg when it comes to our sexuality. But foreplay, what we do with and for our lover *before* intercourse, not only creates the foundation but also determines the quality of the sexual interlude. In the fifteen plus years that I have consciously listened to both women and men, the most significant lesson I have learned is this: the key to fabulous sex is in the foreplay. This is the time when our skills and know-how have the most dramatic impact. And when it comes to foreplay, sexual proficiency begins with the hands.

Hands are miraculous purveyors of pleasure. With more than 72,000 nerve endings, they can create, elicit, and transfer sexual stimulation in many powerful, exciting ways. Our sense of touch is truly one of our most powerful and amazing forms of sexual expression. Beyond that, you won't get AIDS by giving your man a hand job. Why? First, because your unbroken skin is your body's greatest protection against any infection and that includes sexually transmitted diseases. To check if you have an invisible cut or abrasion on your skin, simply run a slice of lemon or a cotton ball dipped in vinegar over the area. Trust me, you'll know in a hot second if you do. Second, you will not get pregnant from a hand job. You could, however, with one of the techniques I'm going to show you, give him the best orgasm he's ever had in his life.

POSITIONING YOURSELF

In order to be able to give him this very special gift, you must find a position in which you'll be comfortable. There's no reason, ladies, to be uncomfortable or cramped into an ungainly posture. The last thing either one of you will appreciate is your getting a charley horse at an inopportune moment. In general, the most comfortable position is for you to be sitting on your knees between his legs. But there are many ways to vary your position and techniques (see below), and I am quite sure that you'll find the combination that bests suits you and your partner.

Here are a couple of seminar favorites:

- Have him sit on the bed, slightly propped up by pillows or on the edge; in both positions you are between his legs.

- Have him sit in a chair with his legs apart and knees bent, resting on an ottoman. You sit on the floor between his legs with your back supported by the ottoman. This ensures your comfort while providing a clear view of the territory you'll be working with.

- Another popular position is on a staircase, (stairs are not as constricting as a bed or chair). You sit between his legs, on a lower step, which gives you more mobility. Put a pillow behind his back or put him at the very top of the stairs. As one travel agent said, "The only stairs we have are in the front of the house, but whatever. It worked like a charm."

Secret from Lou's Archives

If you use saliva to help lubricate, you could risk ending up with dreaded "desert mouth," especially if you've had wine at dinner, which is a natural dessicant.

Remember ladies, you are handling probably the most precious and important part of your gentleman's anatomy. It's doubtful there is another part of his body that so defines his perception of his masculinity. Anything you can do that shows respect for the sensitivity of this area, physically and emotionally, will always be most appreciated. And despite the myth that men have penises resembling "rods of steel," their organs are actually quite tender and delicate, including the skin. This is another reason I am so in favor of using a lubricant either in addition to, or in place of, saliva. I'm not saying one is better than the other, but there is a limitless supply of lubricant and sometimes not enough saliva.

THE PERFECT PLACE FOR A HAND JOB

One of the many advantages of a hand job is that it can be done in a variety of places. Intercourse and fellatio (forgive me ladies, "blow job" just isn't my favorite term), even excessive kissing, are difficult to overlook when being done in public. However, a good hand job can practically be done under the nose of a stranger without detection. It's been known to happen in such places as restaurants (providing the tablecloth is long enough), in airplanes (those little blankets *are* good for something), and on amusement park rides (though you may have to go around more than once). Although admittedly, the risk involved is part of the thrill, by all means, *do* be careful. Being arrested is another serious mood killer. Basically, men are thrilled by a good hand job outside of their bedrooms.

Consider these reported favorite locations:

- stairwells of hotels, libraries, or office buildings
- boardroom tables
- the boss's desk (who knew this was so popular!)
- a restaurant powder room
- laundry rooms
- under the beach blanket
- the kitchen counter, when on your way out of the house for the evening

THE STATE OF THE HANDS

Always keep in mind *presentation, presentation, presentation!* And in the case of manual stimulation, your hands are the center of attention—well, almost the center. In most of the techniques I describe below, you'll be using both your hands, so it's of the utmost importance that they look and feel their best. As I just mentioned, you'll be handling the most tender and sensitive parts of a man's body. Psychologically, he'll make a connection between the way you take care of your hands and the care your hands will take of him.

Needless to say, cleanliness is also key. You wouldn't want him to touch *you* with dirty hands, so show him the same courtesy. You'll want your hands to be smooth, void of any rough spots. For soft, healthy skin, I suggest moisturizing your hands (avoid using perfumed lotions) every morning and evening before you turn in for the night. Your nails should be impeccable and well manicured. The tiniest nick could cause him extreme discomfort. The length and color of your nails are a matter of personal preference, but according to my male surveys, less is often more.

And as for your beautiful baubles: unless your rings or bracelets are perfectly smooth to the touch, I would take them off beforehand.

Techniques

Ladies, you may be familiar with some of these techniques, but I believe the more you know, the more pleasure you (both) will find. Even the world's best chefs don't rest on their laurels after mastering just one dish. They are always looking for ways to create something new using the same ingredients. And in a sexual relationship, those ingredients are your bodies, your attitudes, and your personal style.

In the seminars, we experiment and try out these various techniques with an "instructional product," otherwise known as a dildo. I give all the ladies their choice of which to use. Dildos, which have a base support and come in three natural skin shades—white, black, or mulatto—range in size from 5 inches (the executive model) to 6 inches and even 8 inches long. Believe it or not, most men measure in at 5–6 inches. By the way, most women prefer to practice these movements on something other than "the real thing," and I suggest that you try these techniques at home first. If you don't possess a dildo, a cucumber will do just fine; prop it up in a tall box of tissue to keep it steady. Some women have tried using bananas, but the results were disappointing: bananas aren't nearly firm enough. Going to the green grocers will never feel quite the same again!

All of the techniques require two hands, and are designed ideally with the woman kneeling between his legs, facing her lover. Again, this will afford more range of motion. He should be propped up (with a pillow). I would also suggest that you ask him if he would enjoy watching—men invariably do.

The first technique I'm going to share with you is the now infamous Ode to Bryan. If you recall, Bryan was the friend who first taught me, using a spoon from a cup of latte, what feels best to men.

ODE TO BRYAN
(requires a semierect to fully erect penis)

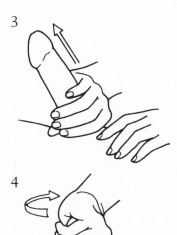

3

4

This is the all-time favorite. A female teacher from Seattle said, "For the first time I was going to make love to him the way I wanted to."

Step 1. Apply the lubricant of your choice generously to both hands. It's a good idea to warm your hands and the lubricant by gently rubbing your hands together.

Step 2. Start with your hands out in front of you, thumbs down. The wrist has to be flexed away from you or you won't be in the position to do the twist, and the *twist is cru-*

5

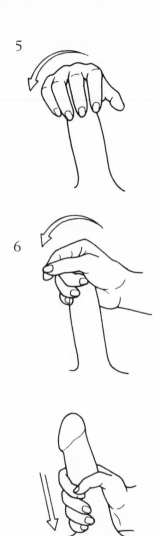

6

cial. Your thumbs are held against your index fingers, they are NOT pointing down like little spikes, palms facing away from you. With one hand (it doesn't matter which one you start with), gently, but firmly hold the base of the penis. Your view should be of the back of your hand and four fingers. His view would be of your thumb, nestled into his pubic hair. Position your other hand so that it will be ready to move into position once the first hand's stroke is complete. Once you have completed one "cycle" both hands will be typically in constant motion, so you need not worry about where they will rest.

Step 3. Maintain the placement of your hand while stroking up the shaft of his penis in a single continuous motion.

Step 4. When you reach the head, twist your hand slightly as if you were carefully opening a jar. Do not twist *until* you reach the head. Bryan's comment was *"The twist is the most critical part and must be done only at the top."*

Step 5. Maintaining as much contact as possible between the head of the penis and the palm of your hand, rotate your hand over the top of the penis, as if you were sculpting its head with the entire palm of your hand.

Step 6. Because of the twist, your thumb will now be facing you and the back of your hand will be facing him. Come over the top and down the shaft again firmly to the starting position and immediately move your second hand into starting position, on top of your finishing hand. NOTE: This is important because you want to have a continuous flow of sensation. You'll get into a flow of motion very quickly. What you want to avoid is the kind of thing beginning dancers do when they count "one-two-three, one-two-three" in their partner's ear.

Step 7. Follow steps 2–6 immediately with your other hand. Alternate hands repeatedly until. . . .

PENIS SAMBA
(requires a semierect to fully erect penis)

The Penis Samba is The Ode To Bryan done very quickly and ONLY at the top/head. And, as you will no doubt discover, this move takes on a rhythm all of its own.

Secret from Lou's Archives

As men age, the intensity and angle of their erections change. When he is an adolescent, his penis is typically close to the abdomen; the older he gets, the wider the angle becomes.

BASKET WEAVING,
OR THE BASKET WEAVE
(requires a semierect to fully erect penis)

4

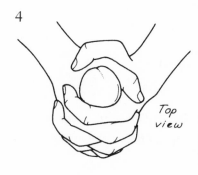

Top view

This particular move was inspired by a woman who suffers from multiple sclerosis. On account of her wrist tiring easily, she needed to use two hands for support. "After the seminar, I went home and did the Basket Weave on him. It was like magic."

5

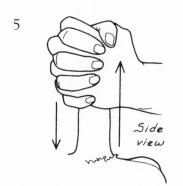

Side view

Step 1. Apply your lubricant of choice generously to both hands.

Step 2. Clasp your hands together, interlacing fingers.

Step 3. Relax thumbs in order to make a hole.

6

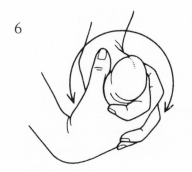

Step 4. Lower your clasped hands onto his penis. The fit should be snug, much like a tight vagina. In essence, you are creating an impostor vagina.

Step 5. Move your clasped hands up and down the shaft, continuing the firm and gentle hold.

Step 6. Twist your clasped hands slowly as they go up and down the shaft, much like the movement inside a washing machine. Use one long twist per shaft length. This isn't a quick swishing back and forth.

HEARTBEAT OF AMERICA
(requires a semierect to fully erect penis)

This technique used to be called the "Pulse" until a woman in a Santa Barbara seminar said, "This ain't no pulse, this is the heartbeat of America."

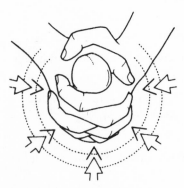

Steps 1–5. Follow instructions for Basket Weaving.

Step 6. Stop the twisting motion and keep in mind that you are imitating a vagina. With your hands at the top of the shaft, gently but firmly begin contracting and releasing your clasped hands, as if they had a pulse of their own, one every second, just as your vagina/PC muscle contracts when you have an orgasm.

Step 7. Keep pulsing while going up and down the shaft. No need to twist while doing this move. You want him to feel the pulse.

Note: You can use a pulse as part of any stroke, and it is particularly good to use as he is ejaculating. You can heighten the orgasmic sensation for him by doing the following:

- Just as he starts to ejaculate and you can feel the pulsations in the shaft of his penis, slow then stop any strong stroking motion (men often become too sensitive to motion at this point).

- Maintaining warm hand contact with the shaft, pulse in time with his ejaculating pulsations until he has stopped ejaculating. (FYI: The pulsing is usually at a rate of one every $8/10$ of a second.)

Secret from Lou's Archives

The "Milking" stroke from the base of the shaft towards the head of the penis that most men use as they are finishing "cleans the pipes" and allows for more intense satisfaction. You can help him with this, as well, ladies. To gauge the strength of the stroke, ask your partner to guide your hand the first time. Your thumb will create the pressure up the back of the urethra.

TAFFY-PULL

(ideal for soft, semierect, or fully erect penis)

Some men prefer this elongating stroke of your hand on his penis, rather than using the strong, compacting, downward stroke of most hand techniques. A male sex therapist in the gentleman's seminar told me this is a stroke that men often use to get themselves erect when masturbating.

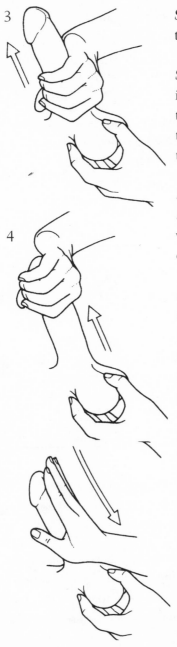

Step 1. Apply lubricant generously to both hands.

Step 2. Clasp the base of his penis in an inverted "okay" sign. Your thumb and finger will be on his tummy, and you will be looking at the back of your hand.

Step 3. Close your fingers, creating a warm soft tube—that impostor vagina. (Your free hand will be discussed in steps 5 and 6.)

Step 4. Gently slide your fingers away from the base toward the head in upward strokes, moving your hand only to the top of the shaft, *not* over the head of his penis. Keep your fingers in contact with his penis on the way back down. Remember, it is important to constantly keep one of your hands in contact with his penis, as any break in your touch will be distracting to him. The stroke can be either parallel to his tummy or in a vertical motion.

Step 5. At the same time you are stroking upward with one hand, your free hand could be gently scratching his inner thighs and his testicles (at no other time will your good manicure be more appreciated). Many men love having their testicles softly scratched and stretched away from their bodies.

Step 6. To further build sensation throughout his entire pelvic area, with your free hand, clasp your thumb against the palm of the hand and use the index finger edge of your free hand like a squeegee stroke going firmly from his belly button towards the base of his penis. I got this idea from men who told me they stroke themselves in this manner with the ends of the fingers of their free hand while masturbating to increase the sensation.

BATTER-UP
(ideal for soft, semierect, or fully erect penis)

This is another version of The Taffy-Pull. Some women report that alternating Taffy-Pull with Batter-Up has led to rave reviews from their partners.

Step 1. Apply lubricant generously to both hands.

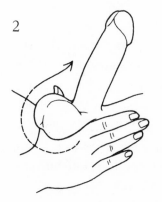

2

Step 2. Cup one hand in a large "U" starting under the testicles.

Step 3. With an open hand, stroke upwards over the testicles. They will lift up with your stroke. As your hand continues up the shaft, the testicles will gently drop back to their normal position under the shaft.

3

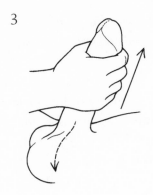

Step 4. Gently slide your fingers away from the base toward the head in upward strokes, moving your hand only to the top of the shaft. Keep your fingers in contact with his penis on the way back down. Again, it's important to remember to constantly keep your hand in full contact with the penis, as any break in your touch will be distracting to him.

Step 5. At the same time you are stroking upward with one hand, gently stroke his inner thighs and his testicles with your free hand.

BASIC ATTENTION
(for soft, semierect, or erect penis)

The main idea here is that a number of men enjoy a firm hold on the base of their penis while they are being stimulated.

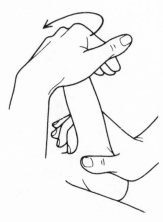

Step 1. Apply the lube of your choice to your hands.

Step 2. Encircle the shaft with the index finger and thumb of one hand, creating a donut; maintain pressure on his pubic area (like a candle holder for the penis). Then, holding the shaft with your fingertips facing him, gently press your fingers into his scrotum with the pinkie edge of your hand; his testicles will be on either side of your fingers. *Be careful not to press directly on the testicles.

Step 3. Use your free hand and perform half of Ode to Bryan on the glans (the head of the penis). Use the relaxed palm of your hand, sculpting over the top.

Secret from Lou's Archives

Men who are not circumcised tend to be more sensitive. Their glans is protected most of the time by the foreskin, except when it's erect, and is thus extremely sensitive to touch.

HAND CROSS
(requires a semierect to fully erect penis)

On first glance there may seem to be a lot of steps in The Hand Cross but believe me, once learned, it's like riding a bicycle. This is another favorite; as one husband of a seminar attendee reported, "When she starts those short up-and-down moves in one place, my eyes roll back into my head."

Step 1. Apply lubricant generously to both hands.

Step 2. Place one hand (your dominant hand) vertically in front of you, fingers up, palm facing away.

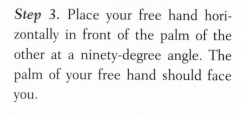

3

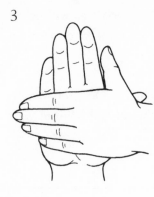

Step 3. Place your free hand horizontally in front of the palm of the other at a ninety-degree angle. The palm of your free hand should face you.

Step 4. Lock the thumb of your horizontal hand unto the thumb "V" of the vertical hand to stabilize your hands, creating a cross with your hands.

5

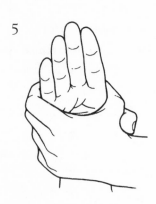

Step 5. Curl the fingers of your horizontal hand around and place the fingertips on the side of the vertical hand, making a tube.

Step 6. It is essential that the fingers of your vertical hand be kept flexed and erect at all times. The important stroking area in this technique is the upper palm, just below your vertical hand's fingers. To give yourself a better idea of how this works, with your vertical fingers flexed back use your other hand to feel the ridge at the base of your fingers across the width of your hand. Now drop your vertical fingers forward at a ninety-degree angle to your palm. Do you see how that nice firm ridge has disap-

8

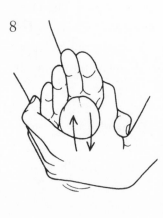

10

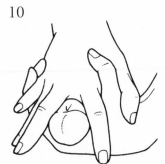

11

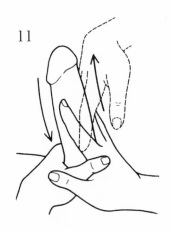

peared? That is why it is so important in this technique to keep your fingers flexed back.

Step 7. With your hands in the cross position described in step 5, gently lower this "tube" over his penis, establishing a snug "impostor vagina" fit with your horizontal hand. This is the hand that establishes the pressure fit in this stroke. *Go slowly.* Your goal here is to mimic the sensation of when the head, typically the widest part of his penis, is first entering you.

Step 8. This is in two parts:

- Start with short, slow, up-and-down strokes, making sure the ridge of the vertical hand moves on and over the frenulum of his penis (the little V-notch on the underside of the shaft, just below the head—this is typically the most sensitive area of the penis).

- Be sure the web of skin between the thumb and index finger of your horizontal hand is gently "catching" the edge of the glans (the head of his penis) as your hands stroke up and over the head.

Step 9. Adjust the length of your stroke by imagining you are on top of him and just allowing the tip of the head of his penis to enter your body. Then vary the speed, pressure, and length of the stroke, mimicking vaginal thrusts. But keep in mind that too much of the same motion at the beginning can cause numbing. Try to vary the speed and pressure of your hands.

Step 10. Every once in a while, let your hands move all the way down to the base of his penis. As you go down the shaft, split the index and middle finger of your vertical hand into a "V," allowing the penis to go between them. Be sure to maintain the gentle pressure with your horizontal hand on the back of the shaft from the tip of the head down to the base. If you have smaller hands, splitting your fingers can be uncomfortable. Don't worry: I know many small-handed ladies who have found they can drop their vertical hand to the horizontal position for a full downward stroke and resume the vertical position once back at the top.

Step 11. Once at the base, reverse the downward stroke by dropping the "V" of your vertical hand so the index and second fingers, which are on either side of his shaft, are now pointing down toward his tummy. Then slide your hands back up to the head of his penis and continue again with steps 2–8.

SCULPTRESS
(ideal for soft, semierect, or fully erect penis)

Imagine yourself as Demi Moore in the movie *Ghost*: you're at a potter's wheel and his whole body is yours to sculpt. Your actual position could be beside, on top, or behind him; anywhere that gives you access to his body. Men often become preoccupied with their designated "sexual" parts, overlooking the other parts crucial to their sexual excitement—specifically, their arms, legs, and torso. Now, with most of your body pressing against his back (remember, our skin is our largest sexual organ), stroke him, while doing The Swirl (page 50).

COIFFEUSE
(ideal for soft, semierect, or fully erect penis)

This technique was discovered quite by accident by a woman with long hair. It got caught on her husband's penis as she was

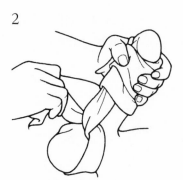

2

changing positions. Much to her surprise, he loved it and the rest is history. You can use your own long hair, buy a wig, or use a velvety or silky scarf. DO NOT use lubricant for this one, unless you wish to end up with helmet head hair or a gooped up scarf.

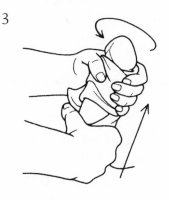

3

Step 1. Position your partner so he can watch what you are doing. The best position is to sit up, facing each other. If you're in bed, place pillows behind him to prop him up. Standing up usually doesn't allow him to be relaxed enough to concentrate on the sensations. He's too busy trying to stand or hang on.

Step 2. Wrap or twirl a large chunk of your hair or a scarf around his shaft. If his penis is not erect at this point, chances are it will be soon.

Step 3. Use a gentle up-and-down twisting motion. Imagine using one hand from Basket Weaving, with your hair underneath creating a new movable texture. To see how this would feel on him, try the texture sensation on yourself. Wrap a chunk of your hair around two or three of your fingers, pretending they are his penis. See the difference? You can also use your hair or a scarf like His Pearl Necklace (page 205). Pull or stroke under the testicles, lifting gently.

FYI: Be careful about knotting silk scarves as often the knots become so tight you can't undo them and you'll ruin the scarf.

TOGETHERNESS
(ideal for soft, semierect, or fully erect penis)

This technique accentuates your awareness of the degree of pressure and the style of stroking your partner prefers. The best position for him is sitting up so he can reach your hands more easily.

Step 1. Apply lubricant generously to both your and your lover's hands.

Step 2. Position your hands one on either side of the shaft of his penis. Have the little finger side of your hands on his tummy, palms facing one another, penis held in between. If he is

2

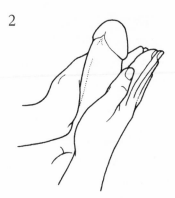

erect, position him in an upright stance; if he's not yet erect, scoop his penis gently up into what will be his upright position.

Step 3. Ask him to place his hands on the outside of yours and guide the motion of your hands. Up and down, twisting, one hand, two? Notice how he moves your hands.

3

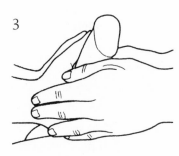

Step 4. Take turns creating different motions and ask which is best. This will help you discover together which technique produces the best results.

Step 5. Continue as you please.

FRUIT IN A BASKET
(ideal for soft, semierect, or fully erect penis)

Those of you who think this technique may be only for well-endowed women—ladies, it is not so.

Step 1. Position yourself so that your breasts act as a shelf for his testicles. You can create this by scooping one forearm underneath both breasts, or placing one hand underneath each breast and holding them up. Position yourself underneath his testicles. The best position is when he is seated on a chair, edge of the

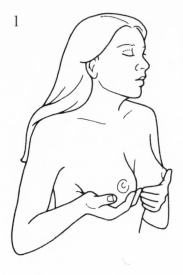

1

bed, or couch and you are seated on the floor below. That way you both are in comfortable positions and have a wide range of motion options.

Step 2. If you wish, apply lubricant generously to your breasts (you may want to use The Madonna lube technique described in Chapter 5).

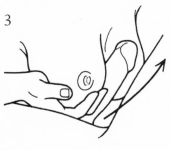

3

Step 3. With an upward arching motion of your body (as if you were a serpent), lift the testicles as if scooping fruit into a basket. Allow them to pass through the channel of your breasts, stroke the glans while cradling the shaft between your breasts, and continue up the shaft.

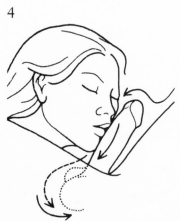

4

Step 4. As you return to the original position in step 1, you can gently drag your chin and then your mouth down his tummy and pass over the shaft and testicles to give him an idea of what might be next. While coming down, you can use your hot breath to accentuate the feeling.

Step 5. Repeat as requested.

PIROUETTE

(requires a semierect to fully erect penis)

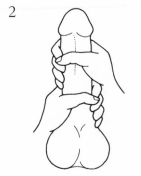

2

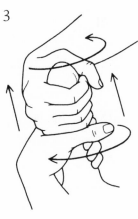

3

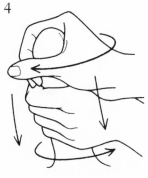

4

This is one of the easiest and most effective two-hand techniques when he's erect. Ladies have also found the Pirouette to be an outstanding combination with oral techniques. The Pirouette is also particularly nifty if the man is standing up against the wall, but be sure you remind him to lock his knees. As the husband of a Texas heiress said, "It's so amazing, it's beyond hot."

Step 1. Apply lubricant generously to both your and your lover's hands.

Step 2. Position your hands, one above the other, on the shaft of his penis, creating a little hand tower. With a closed, warm grip—remember that impostor vagina—you should have the back of both your thumbs facing you. If your man is less endowed, splay the fingers of your lower hand in his pubic hair. Your hands will be moving in opposite directions.

Step 3. UPSTROKE. In the space of one lengthwise stroke up his shaft, your thumbs will twist in opposite directions

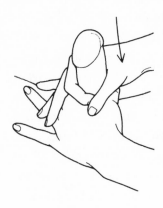

so that your top thumb will go from facing you, to paralleling your left shoulder. The back of your other thumb will be parallel to your right shoulder.

Step 4. DOWNSTROKE. In the space of one warm, moist, downward stroke, your hands will return to their initial positions in step 2. If your man is less endowed, let the fingers on your bottom hand stroke his pubic area.

Splay your fingers and stroke his pubic area

Step 5. Repeat as requested.

Secret from Lou's Archives

You can combine any oral technique with a hand technique. Simply reduce the length of your stroke so that your mouth can stay at the top of his penis.

FIRE STARTER
(ideal for soft, semierect, or fully erect penis)

This one got its name because the motion resembles that of rubbing two sticks together to create a campfire. Good for men with a highly sensitive glans, as the majority of the motion is on the shaft.

Step 1. Apply lubricant generously to both YOUR hands.

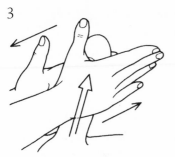

3

Step 2. Position your hands, one on either side of the shaft at the base of his penis. Make sure the little finger sides of your hands are on his tummy, palms facing one another, penis held gently in between. If he is erect, the shaft should be at a ninety-degree angle to your hands, not parallel with them.

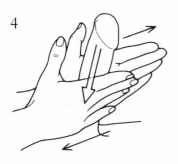

4

Step 3. Move your hands slowly to rapidly in opposite directions. The motion on his shaft should resemble that twirling motion you use on a stick in order to start a fire.

Step 4. Continue from the base of the shaft to the top and return with the same tempo. It is best not to concentrate too long at the top as it may have a numbing effect on him.

Step 5. Continue as you please, perhaps shifting to Basket Weaving.

ONE-ON-ONE COMBINATIONS
(ideal for soft, semierect, or fully erect penis)

This is the "expand your horizons" technique. Essentially, you put one hand on his shaft and the other hand anywhere you or he pleases.

Step 1. Apply lubricant generously to one of your hands.

Step 2. Place the lubricated hand on the shaft and testicles. Begin whatever motion is your favorite.

Step 3. Your free hand will be stroking and building sensation wherever your imagination will lead it. Stroke through his pubic hair with long smooth strokes, use your nails delicately up and down his inner thighs, play with his chest hair, play with his nipples if this is something he enjoys, or pick up his hand and suck on one of his fingers . . . give him a preview of upcoming events.

Secret from Lou's Archives

Whenever you have a free hand, try stroking his pubic hair with long, smooth strokes, trailing your nails delicately up and down his inner thighs. Play with his chest hair, his pubic hair, even the hair inside his bellybutton.

TEMPLE & MITZVAH (OR CHURCH & STEEPLE)

(requires a semierect to fully erect penis)

The key to this technique is the warm sanctuary created within the palms of your two firmly held together hands. The sensation you are mimicking is the penis being at the warm round end of the vagina near the cervix. Due to the position of your hands a very short compact stroke is used. This is a great position for your man to visually enjoy your upper body. Men who love the sensa-

2

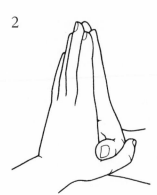

tion of being deeply inside a woman will love this technique. Also, it gives him a great view of your breasts.

Step 1. Apply lubricant generously to both of your hands.

Step 2. Place your hands as if you were praying, palms together, fingers facing upward (not interlaced). For this position remember the "We Must Improve Our Bust" motion women used in the fifties. Your upright hands will be held between your breasts, close to your chest wall.

4

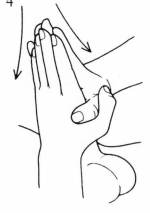

Step 3. Fingers must remain upright and firmly held together. Thumbs cross at the back, facing you, to stabilize your hands.

5

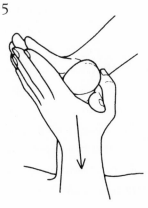

Step 4. You will need to be very close to his crotch to execute this move. Gently lower your hands over his penis, enclosing the head within the sanctuary created by your hands. DON'T drop your hands forward or split your fingers, because in doing so you lose the pressure. Use a firm gentle stroke; you will feel only the head in between your palms.

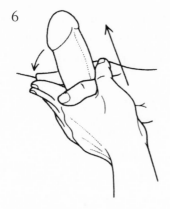

6

Step 5. To elongate the stroke allow the head of the penis to push through between your index fingers and your thumbs. Again, don't drop your hands forward or he will lose the pleasure of the pressure.

Step 6. When you reach the base of the shaft to begin the upward stroke, point your fingers toward his face and start back up the shaft, keeping hands together. You should now be at the starting position in step 4.

Step 7. Continue as you please, perhaps shifting to The Hand Cross.

RAIN PATTERN
(ideal for soft, semierect, or fully erect penis)

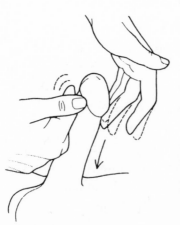

This is a good motion for transition, to keep in contact when shifting position and/or to stay in contact while you slow things down should they should get too excited.

Imagine your fingers are raindrops, mixing a light shower with "gentle" hail. And his lower body and genital area needs watering, lots of watering.

ONE HAND CLAPPING

(requires a semierect to fully erect penis)

This is for those gentlemen who enjoy having their penises or shaft patted and/or gently slapped against something. Steps 4–7 are part of an advanced move from a gentleman who had this done by a woman and said it was the "all time best thing any woman had ever done."

Step 1. Hold his erect penis in one hand.

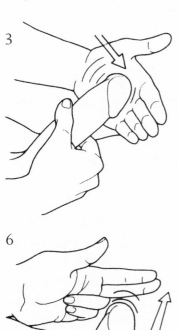

Step 2. If he likes this sensation AND the sound of moisture, consider using a generous amount of lubricant on his tummy or in your hand.

Step 3. Gently tap the glans (head) against the palm of your other hand, or against his tummy gently but firmly, or against your cheek if you so choose.

Step 4. Using both hands, palms facing one another, position your hands so your index and middle fingers are together in an upright position.

Step 5. Position your extended fingers alongside the length of his fully erect shaft.

Step 6. Gently tap the glans back and forth within a two-inch range. Imagine your fingers are a horizontal metronome. (Your piano teacher will never know the usefulness of those lessons). Start with two taps per second.

Step 7. Continue as requested.

SPINAL MASSAGE
(requires a semierect to fully erect penis)

It's not the spine you think.

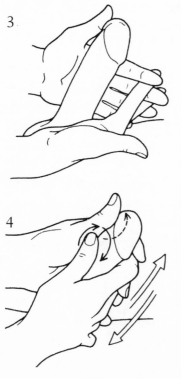

Step 1. Apply your lubricant of choice generously to both hands.

Step 2. Clasp your hands together, loosely interlacing your fingers.

Step 3. Imagine the shaft of his penis is a spine. With your fingers still laced together, spread your palms open and position your hands under the shaft, cradling it with both hands. Your fingers will be pointing more towards his head (the one on his shoulders, that is) than his sides. Your hands will look like an open clam shell.

Step 4. Use your thumbs in a tandem motion as a masseuse would going up your spine. Use that little circular motion, where one thumb circles and crosses the path of the other before you move up.

Step 5. When you reach the top of his penis, clasp your hands together, as you would in The Basket Weave, and firmly but gently stroke all the way to the bottom and start again, opening your hands to cradle his shaft at the end of the stroke.

THE RINGS
(requires a semierect to fully erect penis)

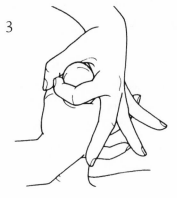

3

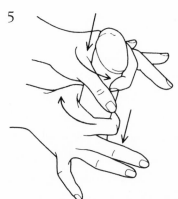

5

This gives a whole new meaning to the "okay" sign.

Step 1. Apply your lubricant of choice generously to both hands.

Step 2. Form the "okay" sign with both hands.

Step 3. With a gentle and then more insistent rhythm, alternate encircling the head of the penis with the "okay" ring of each hand and moving each ring down his shaft.

Step 4. As you approach the bottom with one hand, smoothly slip the other "ring" over the top.

Give That Man a Hand 129

Step 5. Use both "rings" at the top and twist in opposite directions.

THE BIRD CAGE
(requires a semierect to fully erect penis)

A girlfriend told me she learned this one from late night talks amongst her Catholic college roommates.

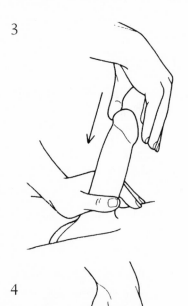

3

4

Step 1. Apply your lubricant of choice generously to both hands.

Step 2. Hold the erect shaft with one hand.

Step 3. Position your other lubricated hand above the head of his penis like an open-hand umbrella. Watch your nails! The ends of your fingers must flare out like the end of a trumpet.

Step 4. With your fingers pointed down and encircling the head, lower your "umbrella" hand in a back-and-forth juicing motion (like you'd juice a lemon on a strainer) down as far as your hand will go until you reach your palm.

Step 5. Juice on the head for a few seconds, then twist back up and start again.

Step 6. Repeat.

TIPS FOR FANTASTIC HAND JOBS:

- Men say the three things about entering a woman that make it most pleasurable are heat, moisture, and a snug fit. That's why warm lubricant and gentle pressure are used in every technique. Your hands are creating an impostor vagina.

- Surveys indicate that Ode to Bryan is the favorite technique for two reasons: the twist sends them into ecstasy, and the upward, elongating stroke closely resembles what many men use to masturbate or get themselves hard.

- Some men are very sensitive on the glans/head area, comparable to those women who find direct clitoral stimulation too much. In this case, it is better to concentrate the motion just below the rim of the head.

- There are no rules about time. If it's been a while since his last sexual encounter, chances are he'll orgasm quickly. Many times a hand job is a prelude to fellatio and/or intercourse. It should last as long as you both are enjoying the experience, until you want to move on to something else, or until the "mission" is accomplished.

- You need to communicate with your partner and make sure you're touching him with enough pressure or force to make it exciting, but not so much that he feels uncomfortable. In the most unfortunate circumstances, a penis literally fractures during masturbation or intercourse.

- If you're at home, keep a towel or cloth nearby. When you're out and about, you may want to have a tissue handy. But remember, most men only ejaculate about two teaspoons of fluid unless they haven't ejaculated in a long time. A seminar favorite is using a warm or hot washcloth: after he orgasms, go prepare it. Then drape it over his entire groin area and clean him up. The warmth and wetness have a tremendous soothing effect and makes him feel very taken care of.

You can't underestimate the power of your hands. And as you'll soon discover, the key to great oral sex comes with the use of a helping hand.

Chapter Seven

Blowing His . . . Mind!

EVERY WOMAN'S GUIDE
TO GREAT ORAL SEX

*"Learning to give great oral sex is a secret
that women have been wanting to learn for centuries.
It is information that women want to know,
and that men love women to know."*

BRYCE BRITTON, FEMALE SEX THERAPIST

AND SEMINAR ATTENDEE

The Greatest Gift

If you've come here first, before reading any of the other chapters, you're probably not alone. I've yet to meet a woman who didn't want to improve her oral sex skills. And who, may I ask, can blame us? If there is one surefire way to put a smile on a man's face, this would be it. And once *you* know and feel that giving your lover oral sex is 100 percent *your* choice, *he'll* appreciate the gift even more.

So, why *do* men love it so much? It's a question I've heard asked more times than I can even remember. Not having first-person knowledge of penises and the psychology that accompanies them, we must go straight to the source for the answer.

(The source I'm referring to here, ladies, is men. In spite of all evidence to the contrary at times, penises don't *really* have minds of their own.) A thirty-seven-year-old male physician put it quite succinctly: "Bad and oral sex don't occur in the same sentence."

There has been a broad range of answers to this perennial question. Some men love oral sex because it makes them surrender. As one man, a stockbroker from New York, said, "I've got my most cherished and sensitive possession in *her* mouth, between *her* jaws and only centimeters away from *her* teeth! If I was ever at a loss of control, this would be the time. But that's *precisely* what I love about it. For me it's about the *surrender* of power . . . for a much greater cause."

There is also a school of thought that believes oral sex isn't "real" sex at all. For these men, oral sex is a way of releasing sexual tension without having to endure the same risks—either physically or emotionally—as intercourse.

But the most common reason men enjoy oral sex is that they don't have to do anything: we women are doing it all for them, so they can simply focus on their absolute pleasure. Your mouth on his penis feels sensational and considerably more personal and intimate. As one man, a banker from Chicago, told me, "A mouth is so much more versatile than a vagina." It's true: we are much more in control of what goes on in our mouths than in our vaginas. In addition, being the visual creatures they are, men find it thrilling to watch the metamorphosis of their penises take place before their very eyes.

Most importantly, I feel, oral sex is the greatest gift of intimacy a woman can bestow upon a man. Between the touch, the sight, and the sound of oral sex, it's almost a sensory overload. Many men have said it's like being in their own erotic film, only it isn't an act and they're starring with the women they love. And finally, they are able to reach orgasm without having to physically work at it. For that reason, your giving them oral sex is truly a gift bestowed.

Once again, I have to confess that I am not now, nor have I ever been, comfortable with the term "blow job." To me, it's a misnomer altogether, as there is actually no blowing involved. There are several theories as to the origin of the expression. The one I give the most credence to dates back to the late 1940s when jazz musicians referred to this act as "playing the skin flute." From there, it evolved into "blow job." Go figure. But as you become more comfortable with giving oral sex to your partner, you'll most likely find the term you're most comfortable with. And for the record, most men refer to oral sex as a "blow job."

There are several secrets I'd like to impart to you on the subject of oral sex. First, the secret to your success and enjoyment in going down on your lover is in *taking control*. Oral sex is a lot more fun for you if you don't have to work so hard. If *you* are controlling the pace and the position in which his penis enters your mouth, there's very little chance of your gagging. You can decide how far that penis goes, and once you've reached your maximum level of comfort, you then simply pull it back out. As his penis becomes less foreign to your mouth, you will gradually be able to take in more of it, should that be what you desire. If you remember nothing else about performing oral sex on a man, let it be this—in order for it to be done effectively, *you* must be in charge. This is something you do for *him*, not something he does for himself *through* you.

WHY SOME WOMEN RESIST
In all the years I've been doing these seminars and speaking to women about their sexual experiences, I've found that there is one obvious distinction between those women who *enjoy* per-

forming fellatio with their lovers and those who don't. The women who like it are the ones who *do* it. The women who don't enjoy fellatio feel it is being *done* to them and tend to shy away from it.

It Doesn't Feel Like a Request

Most often a woman's first experience with oral sex comes at the request of her lover. He'll either come right out and ask to be taken care of, or sometimes just push her head in the general direction of his penis. But either way, she's not going to find a set of instructions down there, telling her what to do. In an attempt to show her what he wants, the guy will usually start thrusting himself in and out of her mouth. For most of us, this does not feel good and certainly isn't any fun. Also, a man usually doesn't know how to give precise directions or describe how and why an action feels good. Indeed, while men remember the best oral sex or manual stimulation they've ever had, they often cannot remember exactly what happened. "I know who it was, I just can't remember what she did," as one man told me.

Gagging

The main reason I hear over and over again as to why women don't like oral sex is that they gag when the penis goes down their throats. Just so you know, it is a very common problem, and make no mistake, giving a man head is very much an acquired skill. Mother Nature gave us a gag reflex as a way of keeping our throats protected. A straight male friend of mine was curious to experiment, using a seminar "instructional product." After attempting several times to put the entire dildo (mind you, this one measured six inches) in his mouth and down his throat, he exclaimed, "How do women learn to do this?" Chances are you're going to gag when performing oral sex; most women do.

The skill comes in learning how to handle the gag reflex. After all, if a woman can be gagged with the proverbial *spoon*, for heaven's sake, what would make her think she wouldn't choke on a man's penis? It doesn't come naturally for *anyone* to have foreign objects plunged down their throats.

Secret from Lou's Archives

The deep throating that many men long for is a result of the porn industry. Let us not forget that most porn films are scripted to appeal to male fantasies. In actuality, it is rare for a woman to be able to do this.

Finding That Hard to Swallow?

The other reason for not giving oral sex to their lovers, women tell me, is that besides gagging, they have issues with swallowing. To swallow his semen or not to swallow it has been an ongoing drama for many women, for as long as people have been practicing oral sex. First and foremost, you should know one thing beyond a shadow of a doubt—if you don't want to swallow, you don't have to. Not swallowing won't make you a bad lover, nor will it in any way diffuse the pleasure your lover receives when he orgasms. A man who makes you believe otherwise does not deserve your gift of oral sex. Period. One woman, a sex therapist herself now in her mid-fifties, told me that she always swallowed when performing oral sex with her husband. For some reason, she no longer likes to swallow and doesn't. It's up to you, ladies.

Whether you want to swallow or not, I think it only fair to tell you that men *do* find it a turn-on to see a woman swallow their semen. More than that, perhaps, they say that being allowed to ejaculate into a woman's mouth gives them an overwhelming feeling of acceptance, specialness, and intimacy. For this reason, it would be kinder, should you *not* want him to come in your mouth, to refrain from using words like "grotesque" and "disgusting" when offering an explanation as to *why*. Imagine how *you* would feel if he were to use words to that effect to describe why he didn't want to taste you.

Secret from Lou's Archives

I happen to have my own personal theory as to why the swallowing of semen can be challenging. First, immediately upon ejaculating, semen gels as a natural buffer against the vaginal environment, so it has a texture some women find unpleasant. Second, it is the nature of sperm to travel *up*hill. The little devils can't help themselves. Swallowing is a downward action, and these guys are doing everything in their power to go . . . *up*.

As a form of compromise, many women allow their lovers to ejaculate into their mouths and then let the semen drip out the sides, rather than swallow it. The Seal and The Ring technique, which we'll discuss further on in the chapter, allows you to use your hand to *catch* his semen and keep it there, without him even knowing it. From his angle, it will appear as if he came in your mouth. There are plenty of other alternatives as well. One woman, an administrative assistant from San Francisco, said, "Just before he comes, I pull him out of my mouth and rub him alongside my cheek, using my warm and wet hand to keep up the contact." A male seminar attendee from New York gave me this suggestion: "My wife doesn't like me to come in her mouth, so right before I orgasm, I lightly tap her, giving her the signal. This way she knows when to pull me out."

The nutritional and caloric value of a man's semen have been debated and discussed for as long as women have been giving men head. Women who enjoy swallowing will insist that semen tastes delicious, that it is high in protein and even that it makes a great facial mask. Women who won't swallow say that semen is fattening and high in sodium. The truth of the matter is, semen contains the simple sugar fructose, and one ejaculation probably contains about 6 calories.

Secret from Lou's Archives

After eating foods such as melon, kiwi, pineapples, celery, or strawberries, men's semen will have a lighter, sweeter taste.

On the other hand, it is possible to influence the taste of semen through diet. The old saying "You are what you eat" has never been more appropriate than when it comes to the taste of intimacy (ladies, for the record, this applies to the way *you* taste, as well). If you *want* to swallow for him, but simply can't stand the way he tastes, don't give up the ship until a change in menu has been put into effect. There is still hope. The consumption of fruits will give him a lighter taste that is far more appealing than the taste you'd get if he eats broccoli, asparagus, or foods that have a high salt content. After eating red meat, semen will be thicker or gummier. Beer and hard liquor also tend to produce a bitter, unpleasant taste in the semen. And needless to say, smoking of any sort (cigarettes, marijuana, cigars, or pipes) will negatively effect the taste of intimate juices (the same goes for you, ladies). In addition, any kind of medication or vitamin can change the taste and sometimes consistency of semen.

If you try a change in diet and *still* find it impossible to swallow, don't beat yourself (or him) up over it. Remember, swallowing is not mandatory, and in fact, only about 20 percent of women swallow during oral sex. This form of oral sex is *yours* and yours alone to give away. If you follow the techniques outlined here, chances are he'll be in such a state by the time he ejaculates, he won't notice or care *where* his semen ends up, he'll only be grateful to have had you there to release it.

The Steps

The second secret I'd like to share is simple: there are five essential elements, each with a degree of variety, to use in creating an amazing oral sex experience for your lover:

THE SEAL AND THE RING

Your best defense against gagging whenever you take your lover's penis into your mouth is to be in control. One of the best ways to assert your control is to use what I call The Seal and The Ring: first, with your thumb and forefinger forming an adjustable "okay" sign, place your fingers around *your* mouth; this way you not only add length to your mouth (the average penis is five to six inches, and our average mouths are only two to three inches). This is known as The Seal. Then, with your thumb and forefinger, tighten and release the pressure, determining exactly how deeply his penis enters your mouth; this is known as The Ring.

If, during an oral encounter, you find that in spite of your best efforts he is too far into your mouth, making you feel as if you're going to choke, try these suggestions for relaxing the gag reflex:

- Stop your mouth motion until the sensation passes, keeping your hand in motion so that he does not lose the sensation and his erection.

- Go on to another move, such as licking or "The Big W" (later in this chapter).

- Slow down and breathe deeply. While he may attribute your deep breathing to sexual excitement, you'll be giving your upper palate a chance to relax.

- Shift the angle at which his penis is entering your mouth. A simple position change can make a big difference. If his penis comes into your mouth straight on, it will go directly to the back of your throat. This would make any woman gag. The trick is to be between his legs and have your mouth come down onto his penis from above. Remember, the object is for you do be doing this to him, not the other way around. If you come down onto his penis, you will have the control necessary to stop it from going any farther than is comfortable for you. No need to worry that he will be making an "L" turn down your throat. The area at the back of the soft palate is very flexible and can easily accommodate the average penis.

By using The Seal and The Ring, you can effectively create a deep throat sensation without having the entire penis in your mouth. One man, a producer of infomercials from the Midwest, described his experience: "My wife is able to take me into the back of her mouth when I am fully erect and I can feel the back of her throat. It is really soft and moist. Then she does the swallowing motion when I am back there. It feels terrific, but not as terrific as when I am soft; when I'm soft, the feeling is ten times more intense."

Secret from Lou's Archives

This suggestion came from a champion fitness instructor who says that when she needs a break while she is "down there," she'll shift the head of the penis from the center of her mouth to the soft cheek area. She maintains the motion, but she can breathe more easily and swallow any extra saliva.

LET THE HANDS HELP YOU

When performing oral sex, you also use your hands. This aspect of oral sex is related to mathematical logic. The average woman's mouth measures approximately two to three inches from her lips to the back of her throat. The average man's penis is five to six inches. Therein lies the dilemma. It is mathematically impossible for the entire average man's penis to fit into the average woman's mouth without some operational adjustments. But there is an easy way to compensate for the difference.

Remember The Seal? While standing in front of a mirror, make your hand into an imaginary megaphone (fingers rounded in a cylinder shape) and hold it up to your mouth. That's the position your hand should be in whenever his penis enters your mouth. It creates the sensation of a tube, plenty long enough to accommodate the length of his shaft while enabling you to monitor, using The Ring, exactly how far the penis goes into your mouth, thereby forming the seal (i.e., your hand should stay *sealed* to your lips).

Up and Down Motion

With your hand "sealed" to your mouth and your teeth covered by your lips or buffered by your hand, move up and down the length of his shaft (or as far as you are comfortable), varying the speed and length of the stroke. You can adjust the amount of pressure on the shaft either by opening your mouth wider or closing it more, cushioned by your lips covering your teeth or, if you find your lips and jaw tend to get sore, use the "ring" of your fingers that are attached to your mouth.

Hand Twisting

The hand that is sealed to your mouth twists back and forth a la one half of a Pirouette motion (see Chapter 6).

Minding the Stepchildren

This is a term of endearment that was used once by a woman in a seminar, and it stuck. In learning about the ways in which to involve a man's testicles, a woman from Dallas said, "Oh, honey, they're like stepchildren, they tend to be ignored!" The fact is, most men truly delight in having their balls played with in the right way.

It's very easy to incorporate a little ball playing into oral sex. After all, you *do* have a free hand. While one hand is attached to your mouth and going up and down his shaft, the other one can be fondling his testicles. What this does is broaden the area of sexual sensation and pleasure. I'm going to give you a few different ways to go about it, but needless to say, it is imperative, ladies, that you tread lightly here. Men are extremely sensitive in this area. Doing it right can provide him with a whole new definition of orgasm. Doing it wrong can produce an entirely different effect altogether, namely, he'll cry out in pain! Remember, they aren't called the "family jewels" for nothing. There are two things to take into consideration before "playing balls" with your lover. The first is whether or not *you've* ever handled a man's testicles before and the second is whether *he's* ever had his testicles handled before. If you've never touched these tender sacs, it is much better to err on the side of gentleness than on the side of strength. The same applies if your lover is new to this experience.

Another place to start is on that soft, hairless skin between his anus and his testicles, the perineum. While the one hand is otherwise engaged, stroke him lightly right there with your free fingers, as if you're motioning someone to come a little closer. Once he becomes comfortable with that feeling (which shouldn't take long at all), tease him a bit by letting your fingers stroke over his balls with the same motion. After doing that once or twice, go back to the area between his balls and anus. He is likely to either tell you to touch his testicles again, or try to guide your hand to them. This is good. It means he trusts you and feels safe. Even so, making him wait for it a little longer will heighten his excitement. You'll be able to tell immediately by his verbal and physical reaction what is turning him on. Even a little pull to some men feels wonderful. Just don't squeeze or pinch

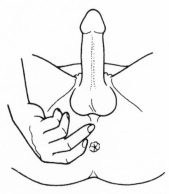

Stroking the perineum

his balls together. One woman told me that her husband absolutely loves to have his balls "yanked on!" Needless to say, at no time is a good manicure more crucial. Not only will he be watching your hands carefully, but more importantly, he'll be able to feel the tiniest of flaws in your fingernails.

Secret from Lou's Archives

When handling the testicles, they should be treated like small, breakable eggs.

Use Your Free Hand

Keep your other hand moving, letting it roam around his body. Try these moves:

- Lightly scratch his thighs or anywhere else you can reach. Alternate swirling and straight strokes so he can't anticipate what's next.

- Be sure to balance the sensation so that whatever motion you use on one side of his body you use on the other.

- Tease his pubic hair with your fingers.

- Play with the "stepchildren" (earlier in chapter).

- Stroke the line from his bellybutton to his pubic bone with your fingertips.

- Using the edge of your hand like a squeegee, create a light pressure wave along the line from his bellybutton to his pubic bone.

Ms. Hoover

How much suction should you use? Due to how our mouths are constructed we can really only suck on the first inch and a half of a man's penis. If a penis is any farther into your mouth, you have to drop your tongue to accommodate it and it is your tongue against the roof of your mouth that creates the suction. Some men have said they prefer less to more suction as the strong constant sucking tends to concentrate all the sensation in the head and doesn't allow for a buildup throughout their entire groin area. Other men love suction and can't get enough. The best way to find out his preference is to ask him to suck on your fingers with the intensity he would prefer and then suck on *his* fingers to see if you're close. Adjust accordingly.

Throat Kegels

This is especially effective when your lover has not yet been aroused to a fully erect state. A throat kegel is the repetitive sucking in of a semierect penis followed by a swallowing motion. What this does (aside from changing his "semi" status rather efficiently) is provide him with the sensation of having his entire penis pulled into your mouth, something that may not be possible when he's in a fully erect state. As one man said, "My wife can take me into the back of her throat when I'm fully erect, but amazingly there is ten times more sensation when I'm soft. She just sucks me in and the pressure of the swallowing . . . whooo!"

There is no question that seeing and feeling your tongue on his penis will turn him on. Use this to its maximum effectiveness. With one hand at the base of the shaft, holding it firmly in place, run your tongue up and down his penis and gently over the head, allowing him to feel both the coarser top side of your tongue where the tastebuds are located, as well as the smoother, softer underside of your tongue. You can even use your tongue as a tool and sculpt the entire length of his penis. Ladies, if he isn't already hard by the time you start on him with your tongue, trust me, chances are he *will* be shortly thereafter.

Tongue Magic

Just as in kissing, the tongue is a crucial part of oral sex. As my friend Bryan said, "Your tongue is always, always, always in motion." Your tongue on his penis can take him to heights of pleasure he never knew existed. Let's try something. Pretending your index and middle fingers are his penis, move them in and out of your mouth, keeping your tongue perfectly still. How does that feel to you? My guess is that it probably feels moist, warm, and pleasant, but a little ho-hum. Now try the action again, but this time move your tongue all around your fingers, keeping your tongue in constant motion as you slide your fingers in and out of your mouth. If you keep the motion going, your fingers are being touched by the top of your tongue, sometimes by the edges of your tongue, and at other times by the underside of your tongue. This creates much more stimulation on his penis and does a far better job of lubricating. Imagine how that difference would be magnified on the most sensitive part of your lover's anatomy.

Lower Tongue Magic

The same kind of "tongue magic" you perform on his penis can be done on his testicles, too. Licking a man's testicles requires some strategic positioning. Lying on a bed, you need to have your face in much the same position he'd be in to perform oral sex on you. To ease access, place a pillow under his hips so your neck won't get sore. Other men in my seminars have suggested you have your lover sit in a chair while you kneel on the floor in front of him. Some men enjoy standing with the woman on her knees in front of him. If this is a position that appeals to you, be sure to secure a pillow to rest your knees on before you begin.

The Big W

There's one move I call The Big W: starting with your tongue burrowed into the area where his leg attaches to his groin, move your tongue (like a writing instrument), in the shape of a large W, going down one side of the scrotum (the sac with his testicles inside), up between his balls, and finishing the stroke on the other side of the scrotum. Then reverse the "W." The tip of your tongue should stroke over the perineum at the middle of the W. In starting and finishing this stroke, your one cheek will have his scrotum on one side and his thigh is on the other cheek. This move has the added advantage of moistening the area with your saliva, so it's easier to take his testicles into your mouth, which is the next move, Tea Bagging.

Tea Bagging

Another mouth move that I've heard men totally enjoy is what I call Tea Bagging. Start with him lying on top and then ask him to get on all fours and crawl over you. Then scoot down beneath him, leaving a trail of kisses on his chest and tummy, then, when your mouth is beneath his groin, place your hands on his hips to guide and lower his hips, dipping his balls into your mouth. Invariably, his penis will harden and do a little bonk, bonk jig against your forehead. If you have enough space in your mouth, try to take both balls inside. But if you can't, don't worry—most women are not able to do this.

Pearly Gates

Some men enjoy having a woman cradle the shaft with one hand and gently nibble up the length of the penis, as if she were eating corn on the cob. One woman said her boyfriend asked her to nibble, bite, and pull, gently with her teeth on the skin of the frenulum (the "V" shaped zone near the head of his penis) just before he came. Initially, when he would tell her to "bite harder," she would worry, then she realized she wasn't hurting him. Another move that involves your teeth is to gently comb over the head of the penis.

Strumming the Frenulum

Here's where you use the back of your tongue, that really smooth area with the nifty ridge in the middle of it, on his frenulum. The sensation is very different from when you use the top of your tongue, or the pointy edges. To get into the proper position:

- Hold the end of his penis under your nose, keeping your chin in contact with the shaft to stabilize the stroke.

- Gently use your supporting hand, which is holding the shaft, to flex the head of the penis away so you have enough room for a nice full tongue stroke, about one-half inch.

- Stroke rapidly crossways across his frenulum with the soft, hot underside of your tongue.
- As a bonus, use your hand to do a half Pirouette stroke (see Chapter 6) on the shaft.

LOOK HIM IN THE EYE

Another secret to incredible oral sex is to make eye contact with him from time to time, provided there is enough light to do so. After all, ladies, you're not there alone. By looking up at your lover occasionally, you're allowing him to see the pleasure *you* derive out of pleasing him. This is also another way of letting him know that you are not only enjoying what you're doing (which will completely turn him on) but that you are in total control, which will make him relax and feel safe.

THE GREATEST GIFT: PUTTING IT ALL TOGETHER

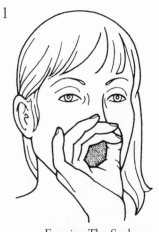
1

Forming The Seal
and The Ring

If you put the steps together, it should look like this:

1. Use your hands to form The Seal and The Ring.

2. Move your mouth up and down the length of his shaft, while maintaining a comfortable level of suction. Meanwhile, use the hand attached to your mouth for the up and down motion and twisting.

2

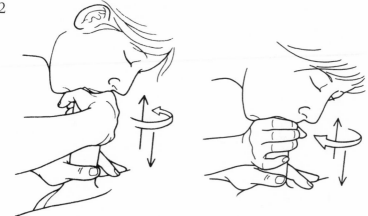

Moving up and down the shaft . . . while twisting

3

4

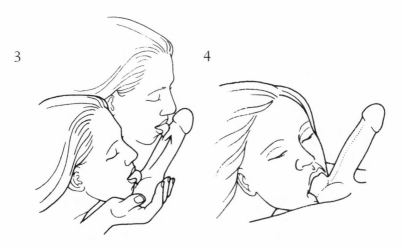

Tongue Magic and
Lower Tongue Magic

Minding the
Stepchildren (Tea Bagging)

3. Keep your tongue in constant motion, moving occasionally to Tongue Magic and The Big W.

4. Don't forget to Mind the Stepchildren, whether you do so with your hands or mouth.

5. Let your free hand roam the rest of his body.

6. Look him in the eye.

VARIETY IS THE SPICE OF LIFE
There are other things you can do to add diversity to the experience of taking him in your mouth.

Tricks with Mints
Suck on a strong mint such as an Altoid, a Halls menthol drop, or a Nice cough drop. Once the mint has begun to dissolve, begin to suck on him. This provides a tingling sensation that many men truly enjoy. Let the mint partially melt in your mouth for two reasons: 1) your mouth will be better coated, and 2) the mint will be smaller and easier to tuck into the side of your mouth. Otherwise you'll be concentrating on mint location, not him.

The Hummer
Another form of tingle, often referred to as a "Hummer," is just what it sounds like. After taking his penis into your mouth, begin a low, vibrating hum. To get an idea of how this feels, once again put your fingers in your mouth and softly moan. As you change pitches the vibration changes, and the most intense vibration is at the front, not the back, of your mouth, where the densest tissue is located. As one woman told me, she can be reciting her grocery list and he wouldn't care—he loves the sensation.

Hot/Cold Shift
Some women have expressed that their men prefer a chilled sensation over a tingly one. The next time you have his penis in your mouth, try moving a few pieces of crushed ice around while

giving him a tongue massage and see how he likes it. A variation on that theme, which can be equally erotic for some men, is to heat up your mouth before having him enter it. Take a sip of hot coffee or tea, swirl it around before swallowing and then guide his penis into your mouth, remembering to keep your tongue in motion at all times. Your morning coffee will never be the same again. Or, with one hand or your mouth on his penis, stroke an ice cube gently underneath his testicles over the perineal area. Be sure to hold the ice cube in a tissue, as you can control it better. It will also absorb any melting. Don't remain in any one place for too long; your aim is not to numb him.

TIPS

- It won't take long to discover that the secret to giving great head is to find your "rhythm," and that rhythm can and will change with each partner, depending on his specific likes and dislikes. What will ensure your success with every encounter is to remember the four different motions you use whenever performing oral sex. When and how you use them will depend on your rhythm, but the motions themselves are always the same.

- The soft palate at the back of your throat is very slippery and has lots of give, unless you are suffering from a case of dry mouth. This can happen when you've consumed a lot of alcohol or salt or are not properly hydrated. It is always a good idea to keep a glass of water by the side of the bed, just in case.

- Once you have reached your comfort level of insertion, allow the penis to stay there for a short time so that you become accustomed to the feeling. Your palate has a good memory. The next time he enters your mouth, you will be able to take him at least as far down as you did during your previous encounter. With a little practice and patience, you'll be able to take him farther each time you try. This, again, is only applicable if you desire to do so. Linda Lovelace is not the role model for all women.

- When sucking, it's best to use short, intense bursts, rather than constant, long vacuuming, which concentrates too much suction on the head.

- Some men who are circumcised love attention to the scar tissue area; one woman quoted her husband as saying, "I thank my parents everyday for having me circumcised. I just love it when you run your tongue around the track."

- Careful about your dental work—and teeth—when performing oral sex. As one woman reported, "I didn't know until the damage was done that I had lacerated my husband's penis with a sharp edge of a new crown."

With these tips, your oral sex experiences are always going to be pleasurable. And though I've said this before, I think it bears repeating once again: the joy you derive out of pleasing him is worth its weight in gold—of that there is no doubt. But knowing you alone possess the ability to deliver it is likely to do more to reflect your power as a woman than anything you can even imagine.

Like all sex, the key to great oral sex is communication—be open to what your partner feels and desires. Men can help you determine what feels best for them, so try not to be afraid to ask your partner to describe what he likes. And remember, when you go down on your man, it is an expression of ultimate intimacy.

Chapter Eight

The Outer Limits

ONLY FOR THE
SEXUALLY ADVENTUROUS

*"When I experienced the benefits of my girlfriend's firsthand
knowledge of these techniques, it was the happiest moment
of my young life. Suddenly colors were more vibrant,
food tasted better, and everything became more vivid.
They can't take that away from me. I felt like I had
stuck my finger in an electrical socket."*
MALE SEMINAR ATTENDEE, NOVELIST, AGE 40

Back Door Misconceptions

I must admit when Bryan of Ode to Bryan fame first told me
about the things to do to a man that are in this chapter my reaction was "You've got to be kidding, there is NO WAY!" His calm
response was "Listen, men love this. And because there are so
few women who know about it much less *do it,* you will surprise
him beyond belief." He was right. What he was talking about
was anal play, manual and oral.

There are those who will feel this is the goldmine chapter
and others for whom it is a foreign country they will never visit.
This chapter discusses practices women typically enjoy and pro-

gressively add to their sexual "wardrobe" once they are either more comfortable with sex in general, or more comfortable in their relationship. From the most practical of standpoints, you need to understand that the anus is one of the most highly sensitive areas of our bodies.

There are also a lot of misconceptions surrounding anal sex. One of the biggest is its association with homosexuality: while many gay men are indeed familiar with the pleasures of anal sex, I have learned through my research that many straight men enjoy anal play. So please, try to resist that outdated stigma. As a female real estate broker from Los Angeles attested, "My boyfriend told me he had never felt anything like it. Not only was the sensation unbelievable, but the mere fact that I was doing this to him made it even hotter. He said he saw stars it was so good."

Another woman told me, "We'd gotten into a rut in our sex lives and wanted to get back some of the magic we'd had before. We're married, so trying new partners isn't an option and when we talked about what we'd consider, both of us were surprised at how much we'd like to try anal things. Just goes to show, you don't know 'til you ask."

Some women also enjoy anal play. In some cases, women, for cultural or religious reasons, actually prefer anal intercourse. They don't have to worry about pregnancy and they can maintain their religious standards and preserve their virginity prior to marriage.

In addition, let it be known that one's openness and comfort level with this, or any other sexual idea, has *nothing* to do with one's skill or prowess. So don't let someone try to tell you "If you were more open, less _____ (whatever), you would do this." This hackneyed attitude mimics that high school pressure technique, "If you loved me you'd. . . ." I might suggest ladies, that if a man says this, you tell him, "Gentlemen *request*—they do not pressure, and those gentlemen typically get what they want."

So, as with any sexual information, if it works for you—terrific. And if not, there are plenty of other ways you and your partner can enjoy yourselves sexually.

First Things First

- It goes without saying that in this section cleanliness is next to you-know-what. The sex acts that follow should only be considered after a shower, hot tub, or bidet; this isn't an after-the-gym thing. As one man shouted to his wife when he entered the house, "Honey, I had a bidet!"

- Should you want to penetrate him anally, watch your nails. Make sure they are short enough by testing them on yourself first. You may be surprised at how short you'll prefer them to be. The end of the nail is important but the critical part is the edge of your nail. The anus is tightest at the entry, so that's where it will feel your nails the most.

- The motions you might like to try on your partner can easily be "road tested" on yourself first. That way you can also give better direction to your partner.

- Because this area of the genitals does not self-lubricate and the tissue is very delicate, you will need to use a lubricant and ensure that it is water based if latex condoms are involved.

Secret from Lou's Archives

A recently evacuated bowel contains less bacteria than the average mouth.

The Three Gems

The anal area is loaded with nerve endings and is therefore highly sensitive. There are three basic ways that you can sample the treats of anal sexual play.

ANAL STIMULATION

The reason anal stimulation feels so good is a matter of biology. To better understand this, consider what the PC muscle (Pubococcygeal muscle) does at the moment of orgasm. The PC muscle is a suspensory muscle, like a hammock, that runs like a horizontal figure eight from the front to the back of the pelvis in both sexes. During orgasm the PC muscle in both sexes contracts in rhythmic wave intervals of 0.8/second. Most women are familiar with the vaginal pulsing at the moment of climax yet unaware that their anus will be pulsating at the same time. Because the anus passes through this sheet of muscle, as it contracts so does the anus.

Anal stimulation can be done manually by inserting your fingers or toys such as anal beads, butt plugs, or vibrators. Here are a few tips:

- Use gentle pressure.

- Make sure there are no rough edges on your toys; use a nail file to buff them down.

- Use different styles of stroking: circles around the anus, or stroking solely across the edges, writing the letters of the alphabet—you can even change fonts.

- Vibration can be added through your finger, a slim vibrator, or butt plug.

- To get the area ready for penetration, try inserting one finger for one minute, then two fingers for two minutes.

- Rather than just leaving your finger motionless in the anus, use a gentle curving in and out motion, with about a one-inch range of motion. The curving motion should go from the front to the back of his body, not side to side.

- To relax the anal sphincter and ease penetration, it is easier to insert a finger/small vibrator or anal beads while your partner is breathing deeply and pushing down slightly.

- Any toy used for anal play must only be used for that purpose. Couples who have sex toys must keep the vaginal and anal toys in different bags to ensure they don't get mixed up.

- Anal beads inserted into the rectum can be jogged back and forth inside the rectum prior to orgasm, or at the moment of orgasm, either pulled out all at one time or individually. There should be a ring at the end of the anal beads to act as a flange so the beads cannot be fully inserted into the rectum.

Secret from Lou's Archives

If you're not ready to "go inside" his rectum, try massaging the outside area with your thumb pad. You will see how much this turns him on, and you never know what you'll try next.

THE MALE G-SPOT MASSAGE OR MASSAGING THE PROSTATE

This is the theoretical male equivalent to massaging a woman's G-spot. Many women know about the perineal "hot-spot" under a man's testicles, which is sometimes called the Male G-spot, or the 'taint. (As one seminar attendee said, "It 'taint the balls, 'taint the asshole.") The perineum is that quarter-sized area between the testicles and the anus that has little or no hair on it. Massaging this area can be done either externally or internally, depending on position and preference. Most men have experienced external but not internal stimulation of the pros-tate. A fortysomething broker from Dallas said, "I'd never had anyone even come near my rear and when my girlfriend pushed my legs above my head and massaged around my butthole with her thumb, I had never felt anything like it. She asked me if I wanted more, and I was like 'Hell yes!' When she pushed her finger inside while going down on me, I exploded. It was so intense."

Your massaging the prostate region mimics and heightens three parts of the male orgasmic response:

1. the contraction and pulsing of the urethral bulb inside the prostate

2. the contractions of the prostate

3. the contraction of the PC muscle

So when you massage the male "G-spot" externally or internally, either before or during an orgasm, the sensations of an orgasm are mimicked.

EXTERNAL G-SPOT MASSAGE

To externally massage the prostate, one of the best positions is to have him on his back with you between his legs. Now this can be on a bed, the floor, or with him on a chair in front of you. With one hand on the perineum, use the other to touch and stimulate another part of his body. (For example, try a modified, one-handed Ode to Bryan as you massage the perineum with your other hand.) Typically, the more sensation you can build throughout the experience the better. The most important thing is that whatever position he is in (knees bent is best), you can easily and gently adjust his scrotum, the sac with the testicles in it, to reach that important spot underneath, the perineum.

Again, watch your fingernails. In this area, do not use any stroke if your nails will be felt. That can make a man very nervous. To see the difference nails make in sensation, try stroking the palm of your left hand with your right hand's thumbnail, then stroke using the pad and the first inside joint of your thumb. See the difference in sensation? Keep that in mind when you are playing in the perineal area. And be sure to use a

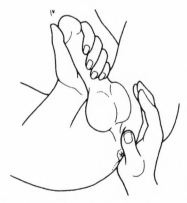

External G-spot massage

light application of your lubricant of choice.

Don't just push with constant pressure against the perineum; after a while the body numbs to constant pressure with no movement. Numbing isn't your aim. An example of this numbing effect: you feel your belt when you first put it on, but then your body starts to ignore it.

Optional Moves for External G-Spot Massage

- Stroke the perineum with circular or straight half-inch strokes, using the fleshy part of your thumb pad.

- Bend your index and middle fingers at the second knuckle. See how they look like little knees? Keep those well -lubricated little knees together and use in a circular motion under the testicles. Stroke in an up-and-down vertical motion, starting at the base of the perineum and continuing up gently between the testicles and back down.

- Some women in my seminars use a vibrator called a Rabbit Pearl, which is designed to be inserted vaginally with a vibrating portion (the Rabbit's nose and its ears) outside to stimulate the clitoris. They report great results by having their partner lying on top of them, the vibrator inserted into themselves with the rabbit vibration on so that it simultaneously stimulates the woman's clitoris and the man's perineal area. The intensity of the vibration can be adjusted by either person.

INTERNAL G-SPOT MASSAGE

Step 1. In preparation, if you so choose, dress your finger with a finger cot or a slim-fitting latex glove. Whether you choose a bare or gloved finger, both should be well lubricated, preferably with a water-based lubricant. Or, use a lubricated sex toy.

Step 2. Insert your finger, or an anal sex toy, very slowly and very gently into your partner's anus. Ask him to bear down slightly as this will ease the entry of your finger or the toy. Let him guide you verbally on when and how to continue. Often it is best to

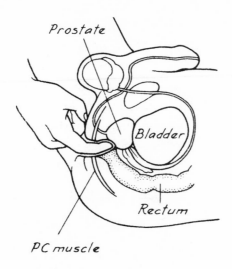

Prostate

Bladder

Rectum

PC muscle

Internal G-spot massage

insert part way and let the sphincter relax, sometimes for a minute or two with your finger (or the toy) remaining still.

Step 3. If you're using a finger, once you are inside past your second knuckle use your finger to give a gentle "come here" signal toward his belly button. You should feel a round sphere. You have found the prostate and are feeling it through the rectal wall.

Step 4. Gentle motion is often the key to enjoying anal play. With your finger still inside your partner, maintain a slow curving in and out motion. Just make sure you don't pull past the edge of your nail. You want the stroking in and out sensation to be from the softness of your finger, not from the edge of your nail.

Step 5. When you are done, use a very gentle, slow motion to withdraw your finger or the toy as you inserted it—be especially gentle after orgasm when the PC muscle has tightened.

For those in the crowd who enjoy giving their partners massages, here is a new twist. A lady in the seminar recommended this as one of their favorites. When he is totally relaxed, recently massaged, and naked on his back, she uses a wand vibrator to massage his back. Then, kneeling on the end of the table and holding the vibrator between her knees, she leans forward to go down on him. The tip of the vibrator, which is still vibrating, nestles into his anus. He goes out of his mind!

Secret from Lou's Archives

Almost any move you make with your fingers can be made by your tongue. With every shape your tongue can assume you can achieve slightly different sensations. To see what I mean try licking the palm of your hand using different strokes and tongue shapes.

ANALINGUS

Here is where cleanliness is imperative. Even though he may be totally clean, a natural scent may linger but will disappear almost immediately when it comes in contact with saliva. However, if your partner has hepatitis, do not do analingus: hepatitis is a nasty virus that is very contagious and this can be one transmission route.

ROSE PETALS
(RIMMING, OR CIRCLING THE WORLD)

For this you will use your tongue like a sculpting tool on his anus. To give you an idea of what this will feel like, run your finger on

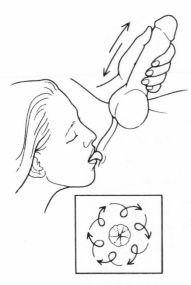

Rose Petals

the inside of your lip. See how smooth that is? The area just inside of the anus feels almost identical. And just like a rose's petals, your tongue should circle around the anus to make a flower.

- You can also draw the spokes of a tire with your tongue, starting with the anus as the hub.

- Push your tongue in slightly; you won't be able to go far, as the strength of the tongue muscle is no match for the strength of the rectal sphincter. He will get a warm, hot, wet sensation.

- Again remember to incorporate other complimentary moves. A favorite among seminar attendees is to be performing Rose Petals on his behind while giving him a hand job at the same time. If he is on all fours, with your free lubricated hand you reach around the front of his thigh and do a slow twisting hand job stroke as you perform analingus. If he is on his back, reach above your head and do a one-handed Taffy-Pull.

- If you wish to heighten sensation try stretching his buttocks cheeks apart. This will expose more of the extremely sensitive anus.

THE BEST POSITIONS FOR ANALINGUS AND MASSAGING THE MALE G-SPOT

- on his back, head pointing away from you
- on all fours facing away from you (you will be behind his buttocks); if he drops his shoulders, you will have an even larger playground available to play with, from his thighs, to his back, to his buttocks, testicles, and anus
- lying on his back, hugging his knees towards his chest so his spine is curved and the anal area is completely available for you to play with

---

Secret from Lou's Archives

If you'd like to try anal sex, seminar attendees recommend using the women's Reality condom, which is made of polyurethene. By removing the adjustable ring at one end, voila, you have the ideal condom for anal sex.

Anal play is not for everyone, but it can add a wonderful dimension to your sexual life with your partner. As with any adventure taken between two people, breaking boundaries can lead to new heights of awareness and, in this case, pleasure.

Chapter Nine

Coming Together at Last

THE MAGIC
OF INTERCOURSE

*"You gave me information that allowed me
to reconnect with my husband and
remember why we got married in the first place."*
FEMALE SEMINAR ATTENDEE,

ACTRESS, AGE 43

You have arrived. Now it's time to learn how to use all that you've
learned about foreplay and push the "last act" over the edge.
Intercourse comes naturally to human beings. It's how we propagate the species. But that's not the same as knowing how to do
it *well*. This chapter will explore the elements of sexual intercourse and show you how to turn the event into a magical experience that completes both of you, transporting you through
pleasure.

This chapter comes late in the book to encourage you to
use all the elements from the previous chapters to enhance
sexual intercourse with your lover. Fast and urgent sex can
indeed be a great rush. However, I have found, in listening to
hundreds and hundreds of women and men, that extending
the foreplay through creating a sensual environment, kissing,

lubrication, oral and manual stimulation, and even anal sex, is what pushes intercourse into the realm of the divine. As a man in his mid-fifties recently told me, "When I was a teenager, I could look at a woman across the room and I'd be saluting the stars. Now she has to walk toward me and sit on my lap." A fortysomething male novelist from Los Angeles had this to say about intercourse: "It's a lot of work: keep thrusting, maintain your erection, push into your toes, stare into her eyes, and say 'I love you!'"

Again, I can't overstate this advice: the factor that most determines whether or not you'll enjoy intercourse is your ability to be an active participant rather than a passive one. Intercourse is an *exchange* of energy, spirit, passion, and love. It isn't intended to be simply tolerated. After all, this *is* the act by which life is created. I'm not suggesting that your reason for making love is, ever will, or should be to create a life. What I am saying is that the act commands respect, for both yourself and your partner. Lying there like a bump on a log while he thrusts himself in and out of you is not a demonstration of respect, spirit, passion, or love.

The secret to having great intercourse is the same as the secret to having great *anything*. You have to be into it. Sex is all about passion and lust and the expression of feelings. It's okay to be noisy. You can scream, moan, talk, or laugh during sex. In fact, in the same way that breathing deeply through a massage helps to enhance the pleasure, many women have said that making noise during intercourse greatly increases *its* physical pleasure.

Granted, if you've always been the silent type during sex, you may not feel particularly comfortable with the idea of turning into a banshee overnight. You don't have to, it's merely an option. Try starting off with a low moan and work your way up. This is not about being loud, it's about being expressive and enthusiastic in your love-life. Of course, if you *should* find yourself enjoying the voice of freedom in bed, it is always wise to be aware of your surroundings. Remember this tip if you're in a hotel or have kids sleeping down the hall—a pillow makes a terrific muffler.

Many women have told me they feel they are adequate but not great at intercourse. If this applies to you, keep reading. I'm going to give you a variety of ways to express yourself in a more exciting and erotic manner than you might have thought about before. I'm going to tell you something again—I know I've said it earlier but it bears repeating: the most alluring thing, according to every man I've ever spoken to about sex, bar none, is to feel as if he's turned his lover on in bed. Men absolutely adore it when they excite us. So if you want to be a better lover, above all else, enjoy yourself.

Female Orgasms

An orgasm is an orgasm is an orgasm. While there are many ways to actually bring on and create an orgasm, there are only a few names to describe them. A number of women experience a tremendous amount of guilt and disappointment because they can't reach an orgasm through intercourse. Let me put your mind at ease. Less than 30 percent of all women climax *during* intercourse! And from what I hear, I think 30 percent is an exaggeration. *There is nothing wrong with you.* Most women can only climax by clitoral stimulation. We've also been led to believe through movies, books, etc., that simultaneous orgasms happen all the time when two people make love. That's not the case: it is *very* unusual.

Many times, women get so disappointed and overcome with feelings of inadequacy about not reaching the orgasm they think they *should* be having, they don't relax and enjoy all the wonderful sensations intercourse *does* provide. What a waste—intercourse can be heavenly, orgasm or not. But there are ways to improve the odds of having an orgasm. For women, it's a question of learning more about your body and how to focus in on certain areas.

Some women make sure they are taken care of during fore-play; others wait until intercourse. Either way, you need to estab-lish open, honest communication with your lover. You must explain to him that as much as you love "doing it," you don't come by intercourse alone. Believe me, he *wants* you to have an orgasm. No doubt this will be even more important to a man who is in love with you, but the truth is, even the most selfish man wants to know that he is capable of making it happen. Men's egos are very wrapped up in pleasing a woman. The worst thing you can do for *either* of you is to fake it. That is the ULTI-MATE form of miscommunication.

Secret from Lou's Archives

According to men, the three most important factors that make entering a woman during intercourse a mind-blowing experi-ence are a combination of the heat, moisture, and pressure.

You don't have to feel guilty about going first all the time, either. Men know better than we do that they are exhausted once they climax. Most of them want nothing more than to curl up next to us and go to sleep afterwards. It's not the same for women. We've got plenty of energy afterwards, and even more importantly, we are left in a state of wanting to give more. It is to their advantage to do us first, and any man with the least bit of sexual experience is well aware of that.

How an orgasm is created can originate anywhere from stimulating the clitoris, to the vagina (more likely from stimulation of the clitoris while being penetrated), to the G-spot, to the breasts, to the anus, to the nipples, and for a fortunate few, their minds—from fantasizing.

Being human, we have to put things into categories, so we want to know if we had what someone else had, and are we normal? So we end up with the categories of where people "feel" orgasms (clitorally and vaginally), but that isn't necessarily where the stimulation was that created the orgasm. Quandary question: If having your breasts stimulated brings on an orgasm felt in your pelvis, what type of orgasm is this? There are some women who claim to even have cervical orgasms.

The solution I offer is, if you have an orgasm from stimulating a certain area, that's a that area orgasm. If indeed you do need to name it. And for those that have a dual origin, you choose. For example, man inserted, woman on top: the orgasm could be from the G-spot being stimulated, or from her clitoris rubbing against him.

Again, though there are essentially three ways in which women can stimulate orgasms, women can achieve and feel an orgasm from many different sources. For example, one female seminar attendee claimed that if her boyfriend sucks on her nipples, she will come. Another woman, a writer from New York, said that often her fantasies can lead her to climax. You just never know what can turn you on!

The three areas for stimulation most often associated with triggering an orgasm in women are:

- the clitoris
- the G-spot
- the vagina (via coital alignment technique)

Secret from Lou's Archives

Most women orgasm only from oral or manual stimulation of their clitoris.

CLITORAL STIMULATION

Non-Intercourse

In this case, an orgasm is typically achieved from direct contact, either from him performing oral sex or by manually stimulating your clitoris using his fingers or a vibrator.

Intercourse

During intercourse, a woman usually achieves an orgasm when she is already stimulated and excited and then gets on top in female-superior position. In this position, she can control the intensity and variety of motions. But as a female banking executive told me, "The only way I can have an orgasm during intercourse is to be stimulated orally, and then I get on top. But if nothing happens within the first five minutes, the bloom is off the rose—ain't nothing gonna happen after that."

An MBA student from Nashville says that when she is on top, her husband often uses a vibrator on her. "My husband holds it in place, and while he's inside of me I rock over the top of it. Not only does he get to see me go nuts, he can feel me come again and again while he's inside of me. He says it's like having his own sex show."

THE G-SPOT

Female orgasms during intercourse without clitoral stimulation are associated with what is commonly known as the G-spot. The G-spot (named in honor of German physician Ernst Grafenberg, who first noted this tissue distinction) is an area approximately the size of a bean, located about two-thirds the length of your middle finger inside the vaginal entrance, above the pubic bone in the front wall. If you imagine a clock overlaying the vaginal entrance, the G-spot is typically at 12 noon. When stimulated, the G-spot swells and enlarges to the size of a dime. For some women, continuous stimulation of this area can lead to a powerful orgasm. For others, G-spot stimulation is unpleasant. And just so you know, there are still other women for whom the much-sought-after G-spot has never been proven to exist at all. The research about the scientific existence of the G-spot is by and large inconclusive for it indicates that while some women have a G-spot, others do not. As one sex therapist told me, "Women should not be held hostage by trying to find their G-spots. Some have them, some don't."

Secret from Lou's Archives

Women who have delivered a child vaginally have a more elastic vagina and the penis is therefore able to stroke and stimulate the front wall, the location of the G-spot, more easily.

The best intercourse positions for achieving G-spot stimulation are rear entry (male enters from behind, woman is on all fours), or female superior, in which she is sitting on top of her partner facing away from him.

VAGINAL ORGASM
(VIA COITAL ALIGNMENT TECHNIQUE)

The "alignment" is between the two parts of the genitals: her clitoris and his pubic bone region. This pubic area is cushioned by the fat tissue so it isn't just hard bone.

Vaginas are mysterious places, known to contain many sensitive areas for stimulation. Some women refer to an orgasm as vaginal because this is the place where they *feel* the most sensation. Sometimes with their partner inside, women find that their orgasm actually comes from clitoral stimulation. Other times, if the man is deep enough inside, and maintains constant contact between her clitoris and his pubic bone at the base of his penis, she can achieve an orgasm via coital alignment technique. This happens most often in the female superior positon or with the man in the male superior position; in both he will be penetrating as deeply as he can. Then she or he starts a slow pelvic rocking motion, about a two-inch range of motion, without breaking contact with her clitoral area. It is the constant contact and motion that brings her to climax.

FEMALE EJACULATION

Some women ejaculate regularly; others, rarely; some, never. Female ejaculation can occur during intercourse, manual play, or during oral sex (cunnilingus). And women who do ejaculate typically know they do, and have had to deal with partners or themselves thinking they have urinated—not so. The source of the fluid is apparently the Bartholin glands, which respond like salivary glands. They squirt, and are located on either side of the urethra, hence people assume the ejaculate is urine.

Men who have tasted and smelled female ejaculate have said, "It has a taste and smell all its own." It has been reported by some as tasting sweet; others say it is little or no different from vaginal secretions.

Secrets of Good Safety

Before I get into the different positions for intercourse, I want to say two words—safety and lubricant. We've already discussed both in great detail so there is no reason to go on and on about them again. Just remember that it is *sexy* to be responsible. Insisting on safe sex until you know for *sure* that you're both healthy and disease-free is a sign of class as well as a show of respect for both yourself and your lover.

Using additional lubricant beyond that which your body produces naturally can only enhance your sexual experience. Whether you self-lubricate or not, no woman stays wet forever. Applying lubricant to him or yourself before or during a sexual encounter will ensure long-lasting comfort. You *know* how painful it can be to have a man enter you when there's not enough moisture for him to slide in easily. It can also cause severe chafing and soreness to his penis, a condition he may not notice at the time, but will most definitely feel later. When this happens, it makes it difficult for him to enjoy intercourse again within a short period of time. The vagina, in its most sexually ready state, should fit a man like a warm, wet, kidskin glove.

Another piece of information to keep in mind has to do with shaving. Some women like to shave their pubic hair because it increases their sensitivity. Please know this can be a bit rough on your man. As one man said, "I was once with a woman who had shaved herself completely. When we were together it had been a few days since she shaved. Man, my shaft was rubbed so raw, it looked like hamburger. But I didn't even notice it until the next morning—by then it was too late to tell her." Waxing is usually more effective, lasts longer, and eliminates rough stubble.

Positions

In spite of all the pictures or drawings you may have seen in countless books depicting hundreds of sexual positions, the truth is there are only six. Everything else is just a variation on a theme. Granted, some of those variations feel incredible and it is certainly worth your while to experiment. There are only eighty-eight keys on a piano, but that doesn't mean people won't continue to create new and beautiful melodies with those same keys throughout eternity. Couples typically use two to three positions during one lovemaking session, moving from one position to another before they finish. Nevertheless, I don't want you thinking that there is something wrong with you or your lover because you haven't had intercourse in fifty or sixty different ways. I am *not* suggesting you have to become a world-class gymnast in the bedroom. You don't have to. While I do encourage variety in all forms of sexual intimacy, the purpose is to push back the boundaries of self-imposed limitations and find *your* ultimate pleasure.

POSITION I: FEMALE SUPERIOR
(WOMAN-ON-TOP)

In the female-superior position, you are on top during intercourse, usually straddling him with the bulk of your weight distributed evenly between both of your knees. This can be done either facing him or facing away from him. Another variation on this position would be for you to squat over him with your feet flat on either side. Many women prefer the female-superior position because it allows for deeper penetration and allows you to control the speed of thrust since you are the person doing the thrusting. It also works well if you are much taller than your man. However, this does require a lot more work on your part and, some say, "ski racers' quads."

Men tend to enjoy this position a lot because it provides them with a good look at your body. They love to see a woman's breasts move up and down with each thrust and see her hair falling or hitting them in the chest or face. Keep in mind that men are visual creatures and they love to watch. A male magazine editor from San Francisco says, "I knew this would be my favorite position from the time I saw a porn film when I was fourteen when this woman in a big skirt lowered herself onto a man. When my wife lowers herself onto me, it takes all my power not to shoot off right then." Men also like to see the expression on your face and know that you're having a good time while you're having sex. A homemaker from Omaha said, "My breasts are unbelievably sensitive, so the combination of me on top leaning forward, while my husband licks, sucks, and plays with my breasts, is a surefire winner."

On the other hand, the women who *don't* enjoy this position say that it's because they feel self-conscious about having their bodies exposed and in full view. If you don't feel particularly confident in the shape or tone of your body, it is understandable that you might feel uncomfortable about having it on display in this manner. But again, according to what men tell me, they are not looking at you with a critical eye at this time. Quite the contrary.

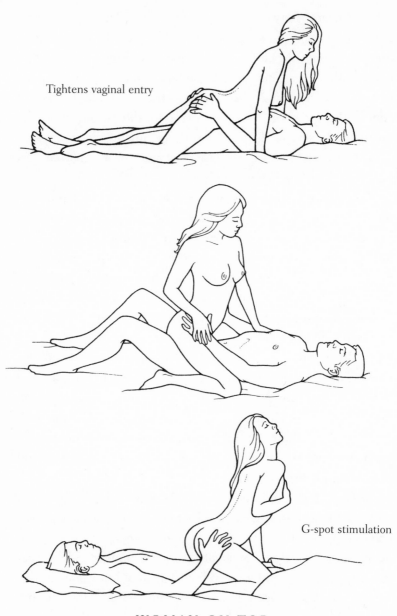

Tightens vaginal entry

G-spot stimulation

WOMAN-ON-TOP

Some men may be critical of women's bodies outside the bedroom, but during sex their women's bodies are beautiful to them. As a Seattle computer executive told me, "By the time I'm with a woman, I want to be intimate with her entire body."

Tips

- To increase the odds of coming during intercourse or coming with him, have your clitoris stimulated to the point where you feel orgasm is imminent, then get into the woman-superior position. If you thrust, there is a good chance you'll be able to reach orgasm with him inside of you.

- Another way to increase the heat between you and your partner is to lower yourself onto him starting at the top of his head, moving your whole body down his body very slowly. Let him see, feel, and taste all of you as you make your way to his feet and then back up to his penis; *then* lower yourself onto his penis. He can also caress your derriere and guide your hips with his hands. You can reach back and play with his testicles.

- Facing him gives you the advantage of being able to make eye contact during intercourse; also, he can be caressing your breasts at the same time you're thrusting.

- While you're on top and facing him, try reaching back with your hands and gently play with his testicles, or try to softly pinch or kiss his nipples. Many men say that having their nipples stimulated drives them wild.

- If you're facing away from him, you will feel him against the front wall of your vagina (the G-spot zone).

POSITION II: MALE SUPERIOR
(MAN-ON-TOP)

This position is the so-called missionary position, the most common position for making love. The woman lies on her back with the man lying over her or slightly to the side of her. Men like it because they can control the depth of penetration as well as the speed of the thrust, according to how far away from orgasm they are. Women like it because there is more body contact than in the other positions. While the other positions are perhaps considered more erotic, this one is the most romantic. Kissing and hugging are easily done in this position and many women say it makes them feel safe and protected.

Tips
- When you're engaged in the male-superior position, there is also a way to involve more of your body than just the genital area. If you haven't tried The Madonna technique (see Chapter 5), you may find this one to be a lot of fun. What you do is sandwich his penis between your breasts. By lifting them up and together, you create a tunnel similar to the vagina. He'll thrust his penis between your breasts

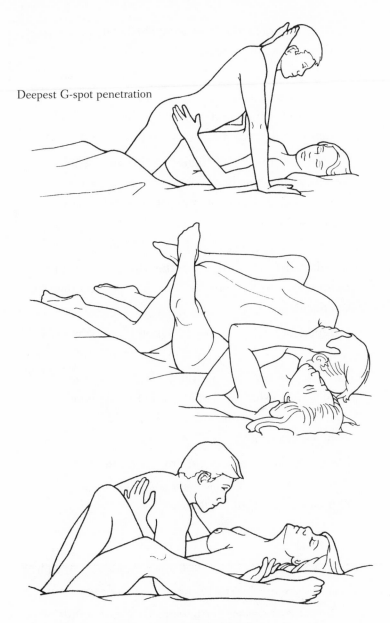

Deepest G-spot penetration

MAN-ON-TOP

and orgasm right there on you. This is also known as "giving a woman a pearl necklace."

- By maneuvering your hands between his legs, you can tenderly squeeze and release his testicles in rhythm to his thrusting. Some men have been known to describe this move as pure ecstasy.

- Massage or insert your finger into his anus while he's thrusting; this has been known to send a man over the edge. (Remember to remove your finger slowly and gently.)

- For men with very large penises, try lying with your legs flat against the bed; this will increase your tightness, as well as prevent him from penetrating too deeply.

- For more genital contact and penetration, wrap your legs around his hips, increasing your pelvic tilt.

- You can give your partner the feeling of sucking him into you by exhaling deeply just before he enters you; then tighten your PC muscle and breathe in as he enters you.

- Place your knees over his shoulders to increase penetration and stimulation of the back of the vaginal wall (G-spot territory).

Secret from Lou's Archives

One seminar attendee says she puts small ice cubes inside herself, then he enters her; her husband loves it!

POSITION III: SIDE-BY-SIDE

For this position, the man and woman are on their sides with their legs entwined like scissors. You can be facing each other or he can be in back of you. The beauty of side-by-side is that most men can thrust for a long time in this position without climaxing. It provides couples the opportunity to make their intimate encounter last. And because penetration is not as deep in this position, women who have lovers with exceptionally large penises say that intercourse is more comfortable for them. Much like in the male-superior position, kissing and hugging are almost inevitable here. A forty-one-year-old male investment banker from London recalls this experience: "Our first time together we had gone camping and slept in a sleeping bag. I'm 6'3" and she's 5'6", so it's easier this way. As she says, sometimes, she can disappear underneath me." Perhaps the best thing about making love side-by-side, however, is that it is the one position that lends itself to falling asleep comfortably in each others' arms afterwards. A sixty-two-year-old award-winning actress says, "I love having my husband behind me. He kind of scoops me in towards him. He has a huge penis, which can sometimes hurt. This way he can have the head inside me and my thighs stimulate the rest of his shaft. After we're done, we fall asleep with him nestled behind me, one arm cupping my breast."

Tips
- With the man behind, he can also stimulate your clitoris.
- Tightening your thighs can increase friction.
- Rear entry in a side-to-side position can be good for pregnant women, as she will be able to support her abdomen and he can play with her, ahem, full breasts.

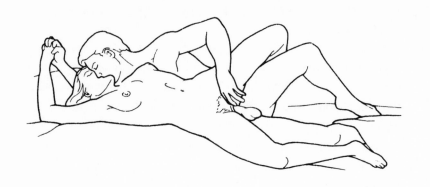

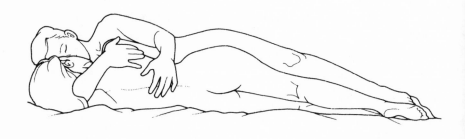

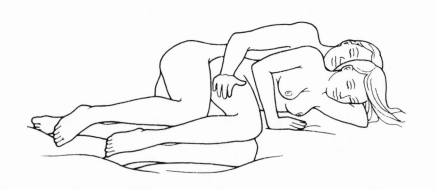

SIDE-BY-SIDE

POSITION IV: MALE-FROM-BEHIND
(DOGGIE STYLE)

Many women have said that the male-from-behind, or doggie-style, position makes for some of their most erotic sex. Men as well find this position highly charged. Their reasons range from the intense depth of penetration to the feeling of taking or being taken. As a dentist from San Diego said, "It is so animal. I love seeing her butt and seeing me fill her up." Another man, a lawyer from Boston, told me, "There is more smell of sex. I not only feel it, I can smell it."

This position can be done with the woman lying flat on her stomach, the woman on all fours, the woman standing up bent over, or the woman lying on her side in front of her lover. The man enters her vagina from the back of her rather than from in front of her. That's why it is often referred to as rear entry or doggie-style.

Tips

- For women who have personal knowledge that their G-spot exists, this is said to be the most effective position for getting to it because of the angle of the penetration by his penis.

- The only drawback to rear entry sex is that because it is *so* highly erotic, men often reach their climax more quickly than they do in other positions.

- Men like to see themselves entering a woman and then banging against her buttocks cheeks. Try putting a mirror facing the bed.

- This position can be painful if you have a tilted uterus or a very large partner.

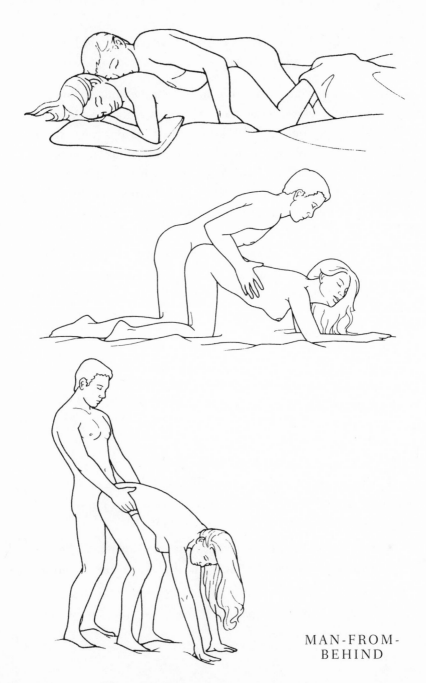

MAN-FROM-
BEHIND

How to Be a Great Lover

- He can be stimulating you with his hands as he penetrates you.

POSITION V: STANDING UP

For the sake of balance, this position is best done with the woman standing against a wall and the man standing in front of her unless he is particularly strong. Though another position is probably best for a long romantic sexual encounter, this one is excellent for hot and urgent sex. It can be done without the complete removal of clothes (a plus when you're both in a hurry) and requires very little space to do it in. Remember the broom closet we talked about in Chapter 2? Well, this is a great position for sex in the broom closet or in the shower. Evidently it has also been done more than once this way in an elevator, because standing-up sex is often referred to as "elevator banging." On the subject of fast, urgent sex, I just want to point out that in given situations most men adore it. It's not that they *don't* adore long, passionate lovemaking sessions, they do. But fast, wild sex in a place that's a little bit dangerous can be exciting. What this kind of sex lacks in romance, it makes up for in heat. There is a certain amount of excitement to be found in knowing that he absolutely *has* to have you, right then and there. It's also very rewarding once in a while to actually *be* the fantasy. Furthermore, men are often so appreciative afterwards of having been indulged, many women say that the next time they have long, romantic sex it lasts *much* longer and is *more* romantic than ever before.

- Make sure that when you wrap your legs around him, you don't cause him discomfort. Take this scenario for instance: "My boyfriend and I were on the

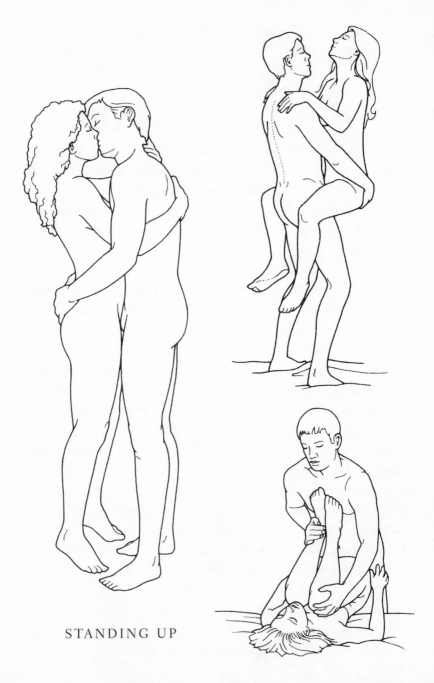

STANDING UP

balcony in Hawaii at sunset. We'd just come in from a cocktail reception and I told him I had on no underwear. He lifted me up on the railing and I wrapped my thighs around him. We proceeded to go absolutely wild, then he started to scream. I thought it was from the passion. Wrong. My stilettos were digging into his calves!"

- Make sure his knees are locked and he is comfortably leaning against a solid wall. As a female twenty-four-year-old bookstore owner remembers, "My boyfriend and I tried to do it standing up with him holding me and I fell backwards because he couldn't lift me easily—and I only weigh 115 pounds!"

POSITION VI: SITTING/KNEELING

Sitting or kneeling is simply a variation of the side-by-side, facing position done at a different height. Many couples enjoy sitting or kneeling because the positions feel novel and give them a break in their routine. Neither position allows for much movement, but they do allow for great face-to-face contact.

Tips
- Sitting, she can be straddling him, facing away while seated on his lap, or facing sideways in his lap.
- He can kneel between her legs and enter her while facing her, while she's seated.
- Either position can help increase a woman's tightness. There is a sharper angle for entry, hence a tighter space.

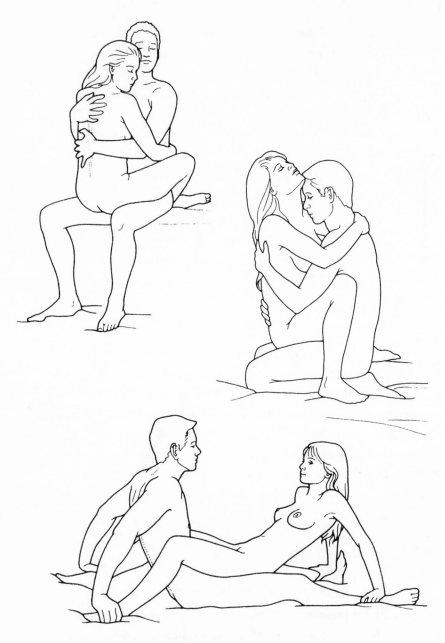

SITTING/KNEELING

- This is an easy position to move to from the female-superior position; the woman just pulls her legs forward and the man can sit up.

- Sitting on a chair is good for couples who want a quickie, or if the woman is pregnant.

Secret from Lou's Archives

With him inside of you, try pulsing around his penis; this not only will increase his stimulation, it may lead to a vaginal orgasm for you.

Vaginal Exercisers: How to Feel Tight

I have been asked numerous times if I knew of any products or ways to strengthen that important vaginal muscle, the PC (pubococcygeal) muscle. To determine the current strength of your PC muscle insert your fingers vaginally, and tighten around them as if you were trying to stop the flow of urine. If it feels like a thin strip closing around your fingers, you need to do some work. If the tightening feels like a broad band you are probably already in good shape. However, if we've had children, and even if not, as we age this is one muscle we want to always have in shape because it is our love muscle. Some men do notice the varying tightness of a woman's vagina. A forty-eight-year-old photographer from Sherman Oaks, California, explained the issue of tightness in this way: "When a woman is tight and you first enter her you can feel her down the whole length of your penis. But then sooner or later, after she's lubricated and gets excited, she loosens up. Other women feel like caves when you enter them because there is no pressure. The tightness is really just at the entry."

The point to remember, ladies, is that while it's probably good for your health and his initial enjoyment to have a strong or tight PC muscle, it's no barrier to his ultimate pleasure. As a male commercial photographer from Los Angeles put it, "What it ultimately comes down to is that the two of you have to communicate what you like and only sometimes is it the marathon stuff."

I cannot stress enough that the inability to reach orgasm through sexual intercourse is not a flaw. Women who *do* are the exception rather than the rule. But this does not mean intercourse can't feel wonderful just the same. It can. Keeping your vaginal muscles tight is a means to that end, and the Kegel exercise for the PC muscle is the best method for vaginal fitness.

The simplest method of Kegel exercise is to regularly squeeze and release the muscles that line your vagina (see below). Just as you would do sets and repetitions of other exercises in the gym, you can do the same with your Kegels. This exercise can be done discreetly while driving, sitting at your desk, or watching television. It won't take long for the vaginal muscles to begin to strengthen. You'll know this is happening when his penis begins to feel thicker and larger inside of you. The tighter the fit of your vaginal glove around his penis, the more sensual the feeling will be for both of you.

Exercise
- Lie supine, knees flexed, feet flat.
- Place one hand on the floor and rest the other gently on your abdomen.

- Contract and internally lift the region between your genitals and anus, squeezing the muscles inward to the center of the body.

- Results are enhanced by breath control: inhale with the contraction and exhale during a controlled release.

- For increased strength, vary the tempo of contractions. Variations include the "elevator," a deep sustained contraction that rises in the body; and "flutters," a series of rapid, intense, surface contractions.

Use your imagination and awareness: try pulsing your PC muscle as you are driving, eating, whenever. Develop a program, start with twenty flutters and twenty big squeezes and then build up. Remember this is a muscle and it will tire easily if not in shape. If you keep up the exercises, I bet you will feel a noticeable difference soon. Here are some other suggestions using toys for tightening this muscle group:

Marble shaped eggs.

These are used in Taoist/eastern sexual technique practices. In the healing Tao egg exercise for women, a marble jade egg is inserted vaginally to assist in exercising the "chi" muscles ("chi" means life-force energy). The chi muscles include the urogenital diaphragm and the PC muscle. Following a twenty-step regimen, you practice moving the egg up and down, side to side, and flipping it within the vaginal barrel. If you are very familiar with your body, have studied a philosophy similar to this, and can contract the top of your vaginal barrel, this could be for you.

Kegelcisor.

A Kegelcisor is a tiny metal dumbbell used for exercising the PC muscle. Approximately six inches long with a ring in the middle, it is inserted vaginally half way up. When you contract your PC muscle, the Kegelcisor provides resistance, as well as indicating how much you're moving it.

Femtone.

Just as a Kegelcisor is a dumbbell for the PC muscle, this is essentially a weight training program using a series of weighted eggs. You start by inserting the lightest egg and work up to the heavier ones. You can keep them inside you while you are walking around. One woman magazine editor, who was also the mother of two, told me, "I figured, 'Big deal. This is so easy. I know I'm in shape down there.' Man, did I get my comeuppance—the weight fell right out!! I then had to start with the number three weight and then worked up to the number five weight."

Intimate Trainer.

The Intimate Trainer is the most high tech—and understandably the most expensive—of the PC exercising items. It is based on the same principle used in physical therapy, where myofibril contraction is stimulated by electric impulse. A European doctor created this chip-programmed vaginal insert, which is about the size of a large tampon, that will stimulate/exercise the PC muscle to do the contracting for you as you rest, sit, or sleep. Originally developed for women with stress (during sneezing) and urge (when they have a full bladder) incontinence, particularly after the birth of a child when the PC muscle is so stretched, it was discovered that the increased strength of the muscle translates into not only increased continence but better sex as well. The Intimate

Trainer is best used when you are still so it doesn't fall out, and it is available in two strengths, six volt or twelve volt.

GENERAL TIPS FOR INTERCOURSE

- If you want to discover the most comfortable or the tightest positions when you are by yourself, get a lifelike dildo and practice in private. Try the different penetration motions and positions and see what feels best for you.

- If you experience a burning sensation during intercourse, check to see if you need more lubricant or if you mistakenly used a lubricant with Nonoxynol-9. If neither of these are a possible explanation, you may want to visit your doctor and check for a possible STD or an allergic reaction to your partner's semen.

- If you feel sharp pain during intercourse, your partner may be hitting your cervix; try changing your position. You may also be irritating episiotomy scars, or again, the problem may be an STD-induced soreness.

- Sometimes the ejaculate will remain inside a woman long after intercourse and come out at the most inopportune moment. If this is something that bothers you, try using a panty liner.

Regardless of how much you exercise and how many different techniques and positions you put into your sexual repertoire, just remember that the single most important factor in determining your level of sexual fulfillment during intercourse will be the release of your inhibitions and the surrendering to the exchange of spirit taking place between you and your lover.

Chapter Ten

Pearls and Other Passionate Playthings

DISCOVER THE PLEASURE OF TOYS

"Why did I never know about these things? They've added a whole new dimension to our lovemaking. It's not that we can't have sex without them. But why should we?"

FEMALE SEMINAR ATTENDEE,

ATTORNEY, AGE 47

What Are Toys?

Typically portable, great as gifts, sexual toys are the items that add the sauce to the entree of sex. One married banker who gave herself a private sexuality seminar for her thirtieth birthday described the information about playthings she got: "I feel like I've opened Pandora's Box and wow, I just don't know where to begin."

We will cover where toys come from, who uses them, how to use them, and the seminar favorites for an Adult Play Chest. Every industry has its trade shows and the adult novelty industry is no different. I attend the Adult Novelty Manufacturers Expo semiannually to ensure I have the latest and newest products available. Even if you are shy or have never used toys before, there may be a toy here that will increase your pleasure and add some spark to your sex life.

All of the following items and products have been tested by the elite corps of "The Sexuality Seminar Field Researchers," who are women just like you! These field researchers are from every demographic group imaginable: female, male, celebrities, non-celebs, executives, non-executives, married, single, straight, gay, bi, golfers, non-golfers, and ranging in age from eighteen to sixty-six. And because they knew their responses would be used by people looking for accurate guidance, they were completely candid about what did and did not work.

Know that for a number of people everything about sex toys can be daunting and nervewracking. Remember, the job of a toy is to enhance, not to take over. There are those who may feel that using toys is entirely too risky—they have visions of horrified relatives finding things in a closet upon one's untimely demise. Whatever your choice, you have to be comfortable with it. For our purposes the discussion will focus on toys and products, not videos, books, or aphrodisiacs, although there will be recommendations and sources at the end of this chapter.

WHO COMES UP WITH THESE IDEAS?

The use of sex-enhancing tools has occurred throughout history. *The Kama Sutra* discusses sexual aids; the Japanese came up with "happy" boxes that contained dildo-like items of varying size and shape. East Indian paintings from the 1700s show lovers using sexual accoutrements, and dildos are further immortalized on Greek pottery and in Egyptian frescos.

The source of ideas for sex toys is threefold. A manufacturer who requested anonymity laughingly told me the number one source of design ideas are the egos of the managers and manufacturing owners. There is a constant need to introduce something "new" via a change in color, shape, or new material. Often, as in the fashion industry, they are knockoffs of another manufacturer's design.

Source number two is ancillary marketing by the porn industry. Product manufacturers bring in the porn stars, typically women, and capitalize on their fame by licensing their names for use on a product the manufacturer then produces, such as the Rayvaness Butt Plug. Fortunately or unfortunately, it's been up to porn actors and the manufacturers themselves to test most of these products. This is where there seems to be a huge gap between the audience they are supposedly manufacturing for and how comfortable that consuming audience is with the products. Porn stars are used to having intimate body parts probed, poked, watched, and vibrated. But most of us know next to nothing about preference, style, size. How do we know how to buy or what to choose? That's where my field researchers came in.

The third source are customers who request that something be created for them.

WHAT QUALIFIES AS A "TOY"?

Just about anything can assume toy status. What we will be discussing are those things used within the "vanilla" mainstream. There are other products for more specialized pursuits and categories such as S&M, bondage, or fetishism. FYI: You do not have a true fetish just because an object, such as leather or spiked heels, turns you on or you really enjoy using them. The definition of a fetish is that you cannot get turned on without that object; it is the object, not the person, that arouses you.

But toys can include a range of everyday items: for some it is a scarf, a belt, a pillow. Should you choose to use things at home all you need is a teensy bit of imagination. Idea: if you really are buying cucumbers for salads choose an extra organically grown (no pesticides), one that tickles your fancy. Be sure it is well cleaned, at room temperature, and chances are your salad making will never be the same again.

We know fabric combinations as great fashion statements—leather with a silk skirt, velvet with chiffon—but they can also be dynamite sensual combinations. Because our skin is our largest sexual organ, any change of texture can be very erotic. Imagine your bare skin feeling soft fleece then cool leather. A velvet or silk scarf can be run down his front and then used on his soon-to-be erect penis. Cushion his testicles with your scarf. Just be careful not to tie your silk scarves too tightly. I would hate to see you take the shears to your Hermes.

HOW DO WE REALLY USE THESE?

Ask. If you are on the phone and ordering from a reputable place (see the list of seminar-preferred establishments in the Sources section at the back of this book), they should walk you through the options before you purchase. Good Vibrations out of San Francisco provides the benchmark for this type of customer service. An editor at *Glamour* who was doing a story on vibrators said, "I've told my friends that buying a dildo from GV is like buying a sweater from J. Crew. Simple, straightforward, and excellent product knowledge by the phone sale staff."

And what if you're in an adult store? It can feel intimidating. Often, people won't establish eye contact and tend to move furtively from area to area. Needless to say, this behavior can make you feel uncomfortable asking about the various toys on display or how to use them. Remember, these stores sell products they are *very* comfortable with; try to ignore the nervous onlookers and approach a sales clerk directly. Most will be courteous and helpful.

Keep in mind that some toys are not intended for use, but are rather purchased as novelties, to be used maybe once or given as gifts. And as my anonymous manufacturing source said, "Honestly, I don't know one manufacturer that uses these things themselves—including me." He further commented that the majority of manufacturers spend their money on the packaging and advertising, not on the research and development of the actual product.

Secret from Lou's Archives

Over twenty years ago, in *Redbook's* sex survey of 100,000 women, one out of five said they used some "device" during their lovemaking and for more than half of those women that device was a vibrator.

Treasures for the Adult Toy Chest

DILDO OR VIBRATOR

These very versatile toys have been around for ages. Technically there is a difference between the two. According to Good Vibrations, dildos are "nonvibrating toys used for insertion—they fill the vagina or rectum, creating a sensation of fullness and pressure that many find highly pleasurable." A vibrator also resembles a penis in shape, but is usually made of a hard plastic material and is battery run. A vibrator's main purpose is to produce vibration wherever the operator wishes it. With the current off, a vibrator can act like a dildo, depending on its shape.

For those who are worried that a vibrator will make you unresponsive to your male partner, do not worry. If you are able to orgasm other ways, manually, orally, or with water, know that this is just another way—often a faster and more intense way. It won't replace your man. Nothing will ever replace men.

Ladies, we know how men have a thing for remote controls, right? Well, there are now vibrators that will allow him to be in the driver's seat, so to speak, when he operates your vibrator— and obviously, only if you want him to. Men have said these vibrators make them feel more a part of her orgasm, as if he was in charge. After all, isn't everything a matter of perception?

Secret from Lou's Archives

For hygienic reasons, before insertion, both dildos and vibrators should be dressed with a condom. It also makes cleanup easier.

Dildo/Vibrator History

Ladies, these things are ancient! The presence of dildos is recorded in ancient Greek, Roman, and Egyptian art; there are also records of French troops giving their wives dildos as masturbatory aids before they marched off to war. In terms of vibrators, according to historian Rachel Maines, these toys were used as early as the 1880s as a medical appliance, "designed to improve the efficiency of medical massage, a task performed since ancient times by physicians, midwives, and their assistants from the time of Hippocrates to that of Freud." Medical and midwifery texts of the 1600s explained that this type of "treatment generally consisted of the insertion of one or more fingers into the vagina and the application of friction to the external genitalia with the other. . . . The objective was to induce hysterical paroxysm, manifested by rapid respiration and pulse, reddening of the skin, vaginal lubrication, and abdominal contractions."[1]

By 1900, "a wide range of vibratory apparatus was available to physicians. Articles and textbooks on vibratory massage technique at the turn of the century praised the machines' versatility for the treatment of nearly all diseases in both sexes, and its [sic] efficiency of time and labor, especially in gynecological massage." Until the late 1920s, vibrators were advertised in women's magazines as home appliances, primarily as an aid to good health and relaxation but with ambiguous overtones, as one advertisement promised, "All the pleasures of youth will throb within you."[2] Maines believes that vibrators fell into disrepute when they started being used for psychotherapeutic treatments and/or when they began appearing in the stag films of the 1920s where their obvious sexual use could not be overlooked. So there is a possibility your grandmama may have been more progressive sexually than you first thought.

Choosing a Dildo That's Right for You

As we head into the twenty-first century there is a style and type of dildo and vibrator to suit every person. Some are completely lifelike, having been molded from real people, often porn stars. Others are disguised creatively. The reason? In Texas, dildos are considered an obscene device, which is defined in their penal code as "any object designed and marketed as useful pri-

[1] Blank, Joani. Good Vibrations: The Complete Guide to Vibrators. pg 4.
[2] Ibid. pp 5–6.

marily for the stimulation of human genital organs." So sex shops sell them as "condom practicing devices." According to one manufacturer of unique shapes, "Most of the unusual dildos sell okay in the Bible belt, because regular dildos aren't legal there, but the people want something they can use, and they like my cacti especially." Who knew?

Most importantly, choose a style that suits you. You have your choice of:

Size:

- Sizes range from very small to full arm size. The larger are admittedly for a specialized "niche" market.

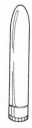

Basic vibrator

Material:

- Plastic, silicone, metal, rubber, vinyl, Jelee (trade name for a soft, clear, often colored plastic)

Shape:

- Straight, curved, lifelike, ridged, smooth, egg, telescoping, and a special design suitable for G-spot/prostate stimulation

- With or without "balls"

- Double dildos for simultaneous penetration for the two partners

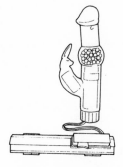

Rabbit Pearl vibrator

Vibrating Features:
- With vibrating dildos, typically the vibrating part will be aligned to stimulate the clitoris while the shaft portion is inserted vaginally. Meanwhile, the shaft portion can be doing something nifty, such as rotating, twisting at the head, or pulsing in and out at the same time the clitoris is being stimulated.

- Power source from battery or electricity

Color:
- Any color you like: black, brown, pink, flesh, clear, purple, white, solids, stripes, sparkles—the list is quite endless

Harnesses:
- Dildos can be used "freestyle" in your hand, or attached to a harness, which is made of leather or fabric and worn around your hips

- Thigh harnesses can be used by either sex when you want full body contact. One seminar attendee told of how her husband, who is paraplegic, fulfilled her beyond her wildest dreams. "He was finally able to penetrate me—I didn't think it was possible." You never know when these toys will work their magic.

How to Use Them:
- Breathe. In any sexual act, breathing is your friend and deep breathing will heighten the sensations.

- Apply to clitoris. Using a vibrator, have your partner stimulate your clitoris—this will add a significant buzz to partner sex. You can cushion the vibration through a garment or the fleshy outer labia. Often women find direct clitoral stimulation too intense until they are more excited. Use a range of stroking motions up and down the clitoral ridge.

- Insert vaginally. Insert either a dildo or vibrator in the vagina; the first 1½ inches are the most sensitive.

- Anally. For those ladies and their men who enjoy anal play, a small butt plug dildo or a vibrating dildo will send you heavenward. Men who enjoy this typically choose a slim little wand style that can be inserted while he's masturbating or while you are manually stimulating him.

- In combination. Use a dildo on yourself or with a partner. This can be accomplished by wearing a harnessed dildo. Depending on design a female wearer may have a vaginal plug dildo in the harness for herself while the "front loaded" dildo is available to penetrate their partner. This way everyone can have the feeling of fullness.

HIS PEARL NECKLACE
(THE ACCESSORIZED "LA COIFFEUSE")

The beauty of giving your lover a pearl necklace is the element of surprise.

I recommend a 30"–36" strand of 8–10 mm round pearls. It's

best to avoid baroque and freshwater bead styles as the irregular shapes aren't conducive to smooth movement, and they could scratch.

Your pearls need to be of good quality, whether or not they are real or imitation. The better the pearls, the better the sensation. Lesser quality pearls won't have a solid enough bead under the pearlizing to adequately pick up your body heat. In this case, heat is a good thing.

Know that you will be using lubricant with the pearls so if your choice is the family heirloom strand make sure you ensure their longevity by having them restrung on nylon versus silk, which is probably what they are strung on now. Silk is hydrophilic and absorbs moisture, which can rot the natural pearl from the inside out—not the kind of thing to explain to future generations. Nylon is a synthetic fiber that doesn't absorb water.

How does one explain the need for restringing? Simple: they are old and need it, or you are a very active woman and you wear your pearls almost constantly, including working out and you've *heard* that nylon is more durable.

Imagine this scenario: dress very slowly for an evening out. Accessorize with a strand of pearls. During dinner, lightly finger or play with your pearls. When you return home, disrobe, and remove all but your pearls.

Step 1. Begin however you like, perhaps with kissing. When you feel ready, undo your pearls and drag them across your lover's body.

Step 2. Lightly lubricate his penis, then slowly adorn him with your pearls, wrapping the strand around his shaft. Be sure to hold the necklace clasp with one finger as you don't want it to scratch and distract him. Because you've worn them out for dinner the pearls will be softly warm.

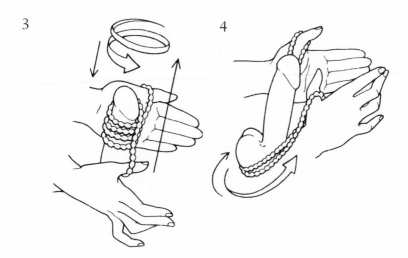

3 4

Step 3. When his penis looks like it is wearing a Princess Diana choker, start slowly stroking him with a Basket Weaving stroke—up and down with a twist.

Step 4. Then unwrap his penis and, as if you are flossing under his testicles, slowly pull the pearls from one side to the other, slightly lifting his testicles.

Step 5. When you are done, "coil the poiles" at the base of his shaft and settle yourself on top of him.

No doubt pearls will start to have a new place in your heart.

Secret from Lou's Archives

If you want to introduce a new form of play into your sex life, and you don't want your partner to know how you got the ideas, tell him "I dreamt it." After all, who has control over your dreams?

SHAFT SLEEVES (THE RIGATONIS)

Probably one of the most versatile and useful toys you can have in your toy chest is the rigatoni. This is a long, 1½-inch tubular sleeve made of a transparent silicone light rubber, with tiny, soft nubbles on the surface. It is available in boxed sets of two or six, all of which have a different texture on the surface. Most men and women are surprised that a shaft sleeve feels so soft. It's also easy to carry in a cosmetic case or shaving kit. With a judicious, not-too-much, not-too-little amount of water-based lubricant (oil will start to break the product down) they can be used by the:

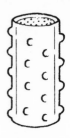

Rigatoni

1. Woman on her partner. Slip one like a finger sleeve over one or two fingers. Some people report using two sleeves, covering different fingers. Apply a light amount of lubricant and use your imagination with any of your favorite hand techniques.

2. Man on his partner, either manually or during intercourse

- Manually: A boon to men. Instead of relying solely on their fingertips to stimulate their partner's clitoral area, men have help in the form of these soft, textured sleeves. Just try one on the palm of your hand. Be sure to put the lubricant on or you won't get the real sensation. Men have reported using two at a time so they can caress and pleasure both sides of the inner labia and clitoral ridge.

- Intercourse: Worn at the base of the penis during deep, slow, penetrative sex. The soft ripples and ridges are able to stimulate the lady. This works for both female-superior and male-superior positions.

3. Solo. Perhaps trying sleeves out during masturbation is the best way to discover the sensations possible with the different textures.

4. On a vibrator. Slipped on a wand vibrator to give a different texture. Care instructions: a little soap and water and they are ready for the next time.

COCK RINGS (THE CALAMARIS)

You may be familiar with cock rings made of metal or leather. My field researchers have said that this softer, incredibly stretchy type is definitely more comfortable going on and coming off, so to speak. The theo-ry behind cock rings is the law of hydraulics: stimulation causes blood to flow in and fill the penis chambers; gravity and a drop off of stimulation cause the blood to flow back out. Cock rings work temporarily by greatly reducing the drop off of penile blood pressure. They do this by holding shut the veins along the sides of the erect penis that allow the blood to flow out, resulting in a firmer, longer lasting erection.

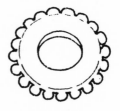

Calamari

Cock rings can be worn during manual stimulation and/or during intercourse. During intercourse some couples have reported they enjoyed starting with a ring and then removing it prior to climax as the pressure became too intense. Others prefer to place the cock ring on while in the middle of sex and finish with it in place. The style demonstrated in the seminars and tested by the field researchers has little nubs that can provide sensation for the partner as well. The scrotum and penis may appear to be a darker color when the ring is in place. This is normal, as there is more blood being held there. The ring should not be worn for longer than ten to twenty minutes without removing it for a few minutes for a break. If he should feel any tingling, remove it immediately.

Directions
- For the cock ring to be most effective, the gentleman or his partner should apply a light lubricant on the ring and the man's penis. It is best to use a water-based lubricant, as it will not break down this plastic like material the way oils and lotions will.

- It's best to apply the ring when he is fully erect, but it is not necessary.

- The correct and most effective position for the ring is at the base of the shaft and underneath the scrotum (see diagram). Placing it only on the shaft can be a problem, some men report. "It was too tight being just on the shaft and even though I thought the other way would be more of the same, oddly, I felt more supported and 'just right'," said one man.

- It is best if the gentleman does the final adjusting over the testicles. Often couples will try a cock ring first during manual play and when they know what works, incorporate it with intercourse.

- Cleanup is as simple as merely washing with soap and water and it's ready for next time.

THE PINK ELEPHANT

This is one of the more favored items ladies buy for their gentlemen. It adds a new dimension to a most favored male pastime, masturbating. It is a translucent pink sleeve that is soft and gently ridged inside—just like us. It is placed snugly onto the erect penis with your choice of water-based lubricant inside, and voila! As one man stated, "In combination with my vivid imagination, three strokes and I was done!" A multipurpose toy, it can be used on him by you, or by himself—either accompanied or solo.

Secret from Lou's Archives

For those concerned that masturbation or "Pink Elephants" will replace you, worry not. Ladies, the majority of men masturbate regularly. Masturbation or the use of a Pink Elephant in no way indicates they aren't sexually satisfied; sometimes, men simply masturbate to relieve a bit of stress. Men have said it is very comforting when they can share these activities with their wives or partners. And some gentlemen enjoy having a spectator.

The Pink Elephant is an ideal "gift" for those times when one is unavailable or your partner is traveling. I have been told it fits well in shaving kits and computer cases. Proponents of the PE are young mothers with children, tired executives, pregnant ladies, and any other woman who wants to connect with her partner but is either too tired or

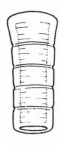

Pink Elephant

unable physically to do so. And if you remember the comment about "sex is hard work," the men in our lives have worn down their batteries as well. One young mother of four, including twins, all under age four, said her husband's original response was, "What is THAT?" and now he says, "Honey, can you get the pink thing?" Says his pleased wife, "This has been a godsend for us."

I CAN SEE CLEARLY NOW

This toy is a clear silicone-like penis sheath with two texturized surfaces, one for the wearer and one for the recipient. ICSCN is worn by a gentleman to augment his width and, to the delight of ladies, its textured bumps heighten her sensation. The idea behind this product is a custom amongst tribes in southeast Asia where they would make a small incision into the skin on the shaft of the penis and insert bells, small stones, pearls, etc., to enhance their ability to pleasure their partners. As a woman from Seattle said, "Oh, weren't they considerate?" There is a lining of soft fringe on the inside for him. There is a slight decrease in sensation for the man. Said one male user, "It felt like a thick condom but I wasn't concerned about losing my erection. The look on her face makes it worthwhile."

BUTT PLUGS AND ANAL BEADS

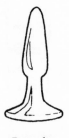

Butt plug

For those who enjoy anal penetration here are the two favorites. The sensation for women is feeling more full, and if intercourse is to take place there is an even greater feeling of fullness. For men, the primary stimulation spot would be the prostate gland. Both toys require lots of lubrication as the anus does not have any natural lubrication.

Butt plugs are in essence a dildo for the anus but with a design adaptation of a flange at the base to ensure it does not fully enter the rectum. It is usually an inverted cone shape so that once it is in, the strength of the sphincter holds it in place.

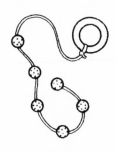

Anal beads

Anal beads are plastic or metal balls all on a string and all but one are inserted into the anus and gently pulled out at the moment of orgasm, as the PC muscle is undergoing orgasmic spasms in the anus.

Care and Cleaning of Your Toys

You should always use water-based lubricants with any of your plastic, latex, or rubber toys because oil will start to break them down and it could result in a sticky, goopy surface. If it says oil anywhere on the ingredients label, it's an oil-based product. See Chapter 5 for field researchers' suggestions on lubricants.

- What's yours is yours and should not be shared. Period. They can bring or get their own toys. This would be the one time your mother's sharing lesson is wrong.

- As with any item that touches your body, or enters your body, use soap and water to clean your toys. If you are using them anally, be sure that is all they are used for, and store them in a separate bag from other (vaginal) toys.

- In order to ensure your own protection, always dress any toy you use with a condom. It keeps you from introducing unseen bacteria into yourself and makes cleaning up very simple. Use hot soapy water.

For the Playfully Advanced

BUNGEE SEX
Probably the most innovative toy I've seen is the bungee sex toy. Designed by a gentleman who loves bungee jumping, this toy allows you to achieve weightless sex. Essentially, it is an ergonomically designed and patented harness system whereby the partner in it can assume umpteen positions for sex while the freestanding or -sitting partner controls the range and intensity of motion. This also provides a most unique way to perform oral sex. The performing partner can move the recipient up and down with just a pinkie motion. Probably the biggest problem with this bungee is locating a ceiling stud to attach it to. It is available in regular or large sizes. For information call Cords Unlimited, 888–828–6433.

REAL DOLL
This takes the blow up doll into the twenty-first century with a bang. It's best I just tell you to find it on www.realdoll.com/ It has too many features and I would do it injustice with a one paragraph description. Suffice it to say this is the doll that Howard Stern had sex with on his show.

Where Can I Get Toys?

There are a number of mail-order, fully illustrated catalogues, as well as stores in most major cities, nationwide, that sell sex toys. Consult Sources at the back of the book.

Toys may not be for everyone, but they can be a lot of fun and add yet another new dimension to sex with your partner.

One Final Word

How to Be a Great Lover is my gift to you. At the risk of sounding sanctimonious, I must tell you that women who have attended my seminars (and their men as well) have said that these techniques have changed their lives. It is my hope that you too can benefit from my long and winding search for useful, practical information about how to become not just proficient as a lover, but a master.

However, keep in mind that the information in this book is yours and yours alone—until you choose to share it. It's personal, private, and special. And no one should feel forced to share this kind of knowledge unless and until she wants to. Remember, this book's premise is that the more information you have, the more confident you will feel as a lover. But it's completely up to you how and when to use the information. If you're in a new relationship, for example, you may want to wait and see how other aspects of intimacy progress before trying a technique. Trust yourself. For those of you in a marriage or long-term relationship, you may have more room to explain to your partner how you suddenly became a sexual master. Again, if you've been with your partner for a long time, you will probably feel more casual about telling him. However, in newer relationships, you may experience some awkwardness when first introducing some of these techniques and he may even wonder how you became such a great lover. Put any worries to rest by showing him the book. In my seminars I have heard again and again women sharing their stories of how they've explained their newfound talents to their men; believe me, the men may be surprised, but they are ultimately grateful.

Above and beyond all, these techniques are meant to enhance your sexual relationship and give both you and your lover a richer, more meaningful intimacy. Enjoy, enjoy, enjoy! And good luck!

Bibliography

Anand, Margo. *The Art of Sexual Ecstasy: The Path of Sacred Sexuality for Western Lovers.* 450 pp. Los Angeles, CA: Jeremy Tarcher, 1989.

Anand, Margo. *The Art of Sexual Magic: Cultivating Sexual Energy to Transform Your Life.* 383 pp. New York, NY: Tarcher/Putnam, 1995.

Bakos, Susan Crain. *What Men Really Want: Straight Talk from Men About Sex.* 225 pp. New York, NY: St. Martin's Paperbacks, 1990.

Barrows, Sydney Biddle. *Mayflower Manners: Etiquette for Consenting Adults.* 221 pp. New York, NY: Doubleday, 1990.

Bechtel, Stefan. *The Practical Encyclopedia of Sex and Health.* 366 pp. Emmaus, PA: Rodale, 1993.

Bechtel, Stefan. *Sex: A Man's Guide.* 500 pp. Emmaus, PA: Rodale, 1996.

Birch, Robert. *Oral Caress: The Loving Guide to Exciting a Woman— A Comprehensive Illustrated Manual on the Joyful Art of Cunnilingus.* 138 pp. Columbus, OH: PEC Publications, 1996.

Bishop, Clifford. *Sex and Spirit: Ecstasy and Transcendence Ritual and Taboo: The Undivided Self.* 184 pp. Boston, MA: Little, Brown and Company, 1996.

Blank, Joani. *Good Vibrations: The Complete Guide to Vibrators.* 70 pp. San Francisco, CA: Down There Press, 1989.

Brothers, Joyce. *What Every Woman Should Know about Men.* 218 pp. New York, NY: Simon and Schuster, 1981.

Brown, Helen Gurley. *Cosmopolitan's Love Book: A Guide to Ecstasy in Bed.* 197 pp. New York, NY: Cosmopolitan Books, 1972.

Caine, K. Winston. *The Male Body: An Owner's Manual.* 405 pp. Emmaus, PA: Rodale, 1996.

Chesser, Eustace. *Strange Loves: The Human Aspects of Sexual Deprivation.* 255 pp. New York, NY: William Morrow and Company, 1971.

Chichester, B., ed. *Sex Secrets: Ways to Satisfy Your Partner Every Time.* 168 pp. Emmaus, PA: Rodale, 1996.

Comfort, Alex. *The Joy of Sex: A Gourmet Guide to Love Making.* 253 pp. New York, NY: Fireside/Simon and Schuster, 1972.

Comfort, Alex. *The New Joy of Sex: A Gourmet Guide to Lovemaking for the Nineties.* 256 pp. New York, NY: Crown Publishers Inc., 1991.

Danielou, Alain. *The Complete Kama Sutra: The First Unabridged Modern Translation of the Classic Indian Text.* 560 pp. Rochester, VT: Park Street Press, 1994.

Deida, David. *The Way of the Superior Lover: A Spiritual Guide to the Sexual Skills.* 131 pp. Austin, TX: Plexus, 1997.

Dick & Jane. *Erotic New York: A Guide to the Red Hot Apple.* 144 pp. New York, NY: City & Company, 1997.

Dodson, Betty. *Sex for One: The Joy of Self-loving.* 191 pp. New York, NY: Crown Trade Paperbacks, 1996.

Douglas, Nik, and Penny Slinger. *Sexual Secrets: The Alchemy of Ecstasy.* 10th Anniversary Issue, 383 pp. Rochester, VT: Destiny Books, 1989.

Estes, Clarissa Pinkola. *Women Who Run with the Wolves: Myths and Stories of the Wild Woman Archetype.* 537 pp. New York, NY: Ballantine, 1992.

Fisher, Helen. *Anatomy of Love: The Natural History of Monogamy, Adultery and Divorce.* 431 pp. New York, NY: W. W. Norton, 1992.

George, Stephen C. *A Lifetime of Sex: The Ultimate Manual on Sex, Women and Relationships for Every Stage of a Man's Life.* 578 pp. Emmaus, PA: Rodale, 1998.

Gerstman, Bradley, Christopher Pizzo, and Rich Seldes. *What Men Really Want: Three Professional Men Reveal to Women What It Takes to Make a Man Yours.* 204 pp. New York, NY: Cliff Street Books/HarperCollins, 1998.

Gordon, Sol. *The New You.* 242 pp. Fayetteville, NY: An Ed-U Press, 1980.

Gray, John. *Mars and Venus in the Bedroom: A Guide to Lasting Romance and Passion.* 206 pp. New York, NY: HarperCollins Publishers, 1995.

Griffin, Gary. *The Condom Encyclopedia.* 128 pp. Los Angeles, CA: Added Dimensions Publishing, 1993.

Hatcher, Robert A. *Contraceptive Technology,* 16th ed. 730 pp. New York, NY: Irvington Publishers, Inc., 1994.

Heimel, Cynthia. *Sex Tips for Girls.* 205 pp. New York, NY: Simon and Schuster, 1983.

Hite, Shere. *The Hite Report: A Nationwide Study on Female Sexuality.* 638 pp. New York, NY: Dell Publishing Company, 1976.

Hite, Shere. *The Hite Report: On Male Sexuality.* 1053 pp. New York, NY: Ballantine, 1981.

Hollander, Xaviera. *The Happy Hooker.* 311 pp. New York, NY: Dell Publishing Company, 1972.

J. *The Sensuous Woman.* 192 pp. New York, NY: Dell Publishing Company, 1969.

Janus, Samuel, and Cynthia Janus. *The Janus Report on Sexual Behavior: The First Broad-Scale Scientific National Survey Since Kinsey.* 430 pp. New York, NY: John Wiley & Sons, Inc., 1993.

Joannides, Paul. *The Guide to Getting It On: A New and Mostly Wonderful Book about Sex.* 368 pp. West Hollywood, CA: Goofy Foot Press, 1996.

Kahn, Sandra. *The Kahn Report on Sexual Preferences.* 278 pp. New York, NY: Avon, 1981.

Kaplan, Helen Singer. *The New Sex Therapy: The Active Treatment of Sexual Disorders.* 544 pp. New York, NY: Brunner/Mazel, 1974.

Legman, G. *The Intimate Kiss: The Modern Classic of Oral Erotic Technique.* 286 pp. New York, NY: Warner Paperback Library, 1973.

Lewinsohn, Richard. *A History of Sexual Customs.* 424 pp. New York, NY: Harper & Brothers, 1958.

Locker, Sari. *Mindblowing Sex in the Real World: Hot Tips for Doing It in the Age of Anxiety.* 258 pp. New York, NY: HarperPerennial, 1995.

Love, Brenda. *Encyclopedia of Unusual Sex Practices.* 336 pp. New York, NY: Barricade Books, Inc., 1992.

Mann, A. T., and Jane Lyle. *Sacred Sexuality.* 192 pp. Rockport, MA: Element Books Limited, 1995.

Massey, Doreen. *Lovers' Guide Encyclopedia: The Definitive Guide to Sex and You.* 256 pp. New York, NY: Thunder's Mouth Press, 1996.

Masters, William, Virginia Johnson, and Robert C. Kolodny. *Heterosexuality.* 595 pp. New York, NY: HarperCollins, 1994.

McCary, James Leslie. *Sexual Myths and Fallacies.* 206 pp. New York, NY: Schocken Paperbacks, 1973.

Morris, Hugh. *The Art of Kissing.* 47 pp. 1936.

Muir, Charles and Caroline. *Tantra: The Art of Conscious Loving.* 134 pp. San Francisco, CA: Mercury House, 1989.

Panati, Charles. *Sexy Origins and Intimate Things: The Rites and Rituals of Straights, Gays, Bi's, Drags, Trans, Virgins and Others.* 526 pp. New York, NY: Penguin Books, 1998.

Parsons, Alexandra. *Facts & Phalluses: A Collection of Bizarre and Intriguing Truths, Legends and Measurements.* 84 pp. New York, NY: St. Martin's Press, 1989.

Patterson, Ella. *Will the Real Women . . . Please Stand Up!* 220 pp. Cedar Hill, TX: Knowledge Concepts, 1993.

Penney, Alexandra. *The Sexiest Sex of All.* 145 pp. New York, NY: Dell Publishing Company, 1993.

Purvis, Kenneth. *The Male Sexual Machine: An Owner's Manual.* 210 pp. New York, NY: St. Martin's Press, 1992.

Reinsch, Judith. *The Kinsey Institute New Report on Sex: What You Must Know to Be Sexually Literate.* 540 pp. New York, NY: St. Martin's Press, 1990.

Rubin, Harriet. *The Princessa: Machiavelli for Women.* 190 pp. New York, NY: Dell Trade Paperback, 1997.

SARK. *Succulent Wild Woman: Dancing with Your Wonder-full Self!* 180 pp. New York, NY: Fireside/Simon & Schuster, 1997.

Schnarch, David. *Passionate Couples: Love, Sex and Intimacy in Emotionally Committed Relationships.* 432 pp. New York, NY: W. W. Norton, 1997.

Schulz, Mona Lisa. *Awakening Intuition: Using Your Mind–Body Network for Insight and Healing.* 398 pp. New York, NY: Harmony Books, 1998.

Shepsut, Asia. *Journey of the Priestess: The Priestess Traditions of the Ancient World—A Spiritual Awakening and Empowerment.* 251 pp. San Francisco, CA: Aquarian/Thorsons, 1993.

Smith, David, and Mike Gordon. *Strange but True Facts about Sex: The Illustrated Book of Sexual Trivia.* 64 pp. Deephaven, MN: Meadowbook Press, 1989.

Stoppard, Miriam. *The Magic of Sex: The Book That Really Tells Men about Women and Women about Men.* 256 pp. New York, NY: Dorling Kindersley, Inc., 1991.

Tannahill, Reay. *Sex in History.* 480 pp. New York, NY: Scarborough House/Briarcliff Manor, 1980.

Taormino, Tristan. *The Ultimate Guide to Anal Sex for Women.* 151 pp. San Francisco, CA: Cleis Press, 1998.

Taylor, Timothy. *The Prehistory of Sex: Four Million Years of Human Sexual Culture.* 356 pp. New York, NY: Bantam, 1996.

Trager, James. *The Women's Chronology: A Year-by-Year Record, from Prehistory to the Present.* 787 pp. New York, NY: Henry Holt, 1994.

Tuleja, Tad. *Curious Customs: The Stories Behind 296 Popular America Rituals*. 210 pp. New York, NY: Harmony Books/Crown, 1987.

Walker, Morton. *Foods for Fabulous Sex: Natural Sexual Nutrients to Trigger Passion, Heighten Response, Improve Performance, & Overcome Dysfunction*. 160 pp. McKinney, TX: Magni Group, 1992.

Watson, Cynthia Mervis. *Love Potions: A Guide to Aphrodisiacs and Sexual Pleasures*. 272 pp. New York, NY: Tarcher/Putnam, 1993.

Welch, Leslee. *Sex Facts: A Handbook for the Carnally Curious*. 100 pp. New York, NY: Carol Publishing, 1992.

Wildwood, Chrissie. *Erotic Aromatherapy: Essential Oils for Lovers*. 160 pp. New York, NY: Sterling Publishing Co., 1994.

Zilbergeld, Bernie. *Male Sexuality*. 411 pp. New York, NY: Bantam Books, 1978.

Zilbergeld, Bernie. *New Male Sexuality: The Truth About Men, Sex and Pleasure*. 580 pp. New York, NY: Bantam Books, 1992.

Zimet, Susan, and Victor Goodman. 121 pp. *The Great Cover-Up: A Condom Compendium*. New Paltz, NY: Civan Inc., 1988.

Sources

WHERE YOU CAN GET THE TOYS

In collecting the best sources for toy products, I asked store owners several questions in order to verify their commitment to high quality products and service, and determine whether they had an open, encouraging attitude. Did they have a positive attitude about sex? Would a woman be comfortable going into the store by herself or ordering over the phone? How big was its selection? Did other companies have access to their mailing list? Was their e-mail site secure?

Stores and Catalogues for Adult Products

WEST COAST

Seattle

Toys in Babeland
707 East Pike Street, Seattle, WA 98122
1–206–328–2914
Catalogue available; order 1–800–658–9119
e-mail: biglove@babeland.com
Web site: www.babeland.com

This is a female-run store, originally created as a place for women and dedicated to their comfort. It now carries some male-oriented products as well.

San Francisco

Good Vibrations
Retail stores: 1210 Valencia Street,
San Francisco, CA 94110
2504 San Pablo Avenue, Berkeley, CA 94702
Mail order: 938 Howard Street, Suite 101,
San Francisco, CA 94103
1–800–BUYVIBE (289-8423) in the U.S. and Canada
415–974–8990; 415–974–8989 fax
e-mail: goodvibe@well.com
Web site: www.goodvibes.com

Good Vibrations is one of the best all-around store/catalogue combinations. Their specialty is vibrators—and they have an almost endless supply and selection. They also offer a vast array of lubricants, special massage oils, videos, and books. The selection of toys and leather goods boasts high quality, durability, and inventive styling. All their products have passed customer satisfaction tests. The staff is known for their courteous, nonjudgmental, sex-positive attitude, and they offer sensitive, knowledgeable, and helpful service.

Los Angeles

The Pleasure Chest (There are three recommended locations for stores bearing this name—the others are in New York and Chicago).

7733 Santa Monica Blvd. 90046
323–650–1022; 323–650–1176 fax
1–800–753–4536 order line
Web site: www.thepleasurechest.com

This Pleasure Chest targets a primarily gay male clientele, with a strong leather focus, though straight men and women may find some interesting, curious toys here.

Condomania
7306 Melrose, Los Angeles, CA 90046
323–933–7865 or 800–9condom (U.S. only)
323–930–5330 for mail ordering outside the U.S.
323–934–9784 fax
Web site: www.condomania.com

This phone/mail-order service is one of the best stores for ordering condoms by mail. They offer a selection of over three hundred different condoms. The e-mail site is secure.

The Love Boutique—two stores
18637 Ventura Blvd., Tarzana, CA 91356
818–342–2400
2924 Wilshire Blvd., Santa Monica, CA 90403
310–453–3459

The two stores are female owned and operated and open seven days a week. While they offer a smaller selection of items, the customer is treated with care by a knowledgeable staff that focuses on making women feel more at ease and comfortable with their sexuality.

San Diego

F Street Stores—ten stores in the San Diego area
751 Fourth Avenue, San Diego 92101; 619–236–0841
2004 University Avenue, San Diego 92104; 619–298–2644
7998 Miramar Road, San Diego 92126; 619–549–8014
1141 Third Avenue, Chula Vista 92011; 619–585–3314
237 East Grand, Escondido 92023; 619–480–6031

The stores in this chain offer a wide range of male and female products. It was also one of the first to create a women's novelty section.

Condoms Plus
1220 University Avenue, San Diego 92103 619–291–7400

This is a general license store for all sorts of gifts as well as condoms. In other words, you can buy a stuffed animal for your child as well as an adult novelty item for your husband. The novelties, however, are in their own section of the store.

MIDWEST

Chicago

The Pleasure Chest (affiliated with the store in New York)
3155 North Broadway, Chicago, IL 60657
773–525–7151
1–800–316–9222 catalogue sales
(same number as for the New York store)

This is the store that defines what an adult store should be like; clean, bright, tastefully presented, with nonjudgmental sales people that look like you and me. This and the New York store (see below) show the impact of being run and operated by the owner, who focuses on taking good care of the customers, the majority of whom are women and couples.

Frenchy's
872 N. State Street, Chicago, IL 60611
312–337–9190

This store has just undergone a major renovation in appearance and size. It is now three times larger and offers a wide range of products for both men and women.

Minneapolis/St. Paul

Fantasy House Gifts—this chain has ten stores in the area
716 West Lake Street
Minneapolis, MN 55408
612–824–2459
Web site: www.fantasygifts.com

Eight stores in Bloomington, Bernsville, St. Louis Park, Crystal, Fridley, Coon Rapids, St. Paul, and two stores in New Jersey, Marlion, and Turnersville. Adult material and novelties presented with a comfortable Midwest environment and attitude. They recently added the Condom Kingdom store in Minneapolis to their operation.

Oklahoma

> Christie's Toy Box
> 1184 N. MacArthur Blvd., Oklahoma City, OK 73127
> 405–942–4622
>
> Christie's is part of a chain of adult stores, ranked #1 in the state of Oklahoma. Stores also exist in Texas.

EAST COAST

New York

> The Pleasure Chest
> 156 Seventh Avenue South (between Charles and Perry)
> New York, NY 10014
> 212–242–4185
> 1–800–643–1025 direct to New York store customer service
> 1–800–316–9222 catalogue sales
> e-mail: apleasurechest.com
> Web site: www.apleasurechest.com
>
> The New York Pleasure Chest and its Chicago sister store are popular, classy, and well-stocked, with a range of products for both men and women, straight and gay.

> Eve's Garden
> 119 West 57th Street, Suite 1201, New York, NY 10019
> 212–757–8651
> 1–800–848–3837 order line
> Web site: www.evesgarden.com

This is a female-owned and operated store. What the Pleasure Chest did in 1972 for gay male consumers Eve's Garden did for women in 1974. Located in the heart of midtown Manhattan, Eve's Garden is in the least likely of areas. It's known far and wide as the matriarch of feminine-focused, sex-positive merchandising.

Condomania—New York
351 Bleecker St., New York, NY 10014
212–691–9442
1–800–9CONDOM U.S. national order line
323–930-5330 for ordering outside the U.S.
213–934–9784 fax
Web site: www.condomania.com

This is probably the best national source for ordering condoms by mail or phone, or on-line. Their Web site is secure and the store itself is friendly and filled with useful novelty items.

North Carolina

Adam & Eve
P.O. Box 800, Carrboro, NC 27510
1–800–765–ADAM (2326)
919–644–1212 customer service

This is the biggest mail-order company in the U.S. that offers a full range of adult novelty products.

CANADA

Toronto

Seduction
577 Yonge Street, Toronto, Ontario, Canada M4Y 1Z2
416–966–6969

This recently opened retail operation is the largest adult
novelty store in North America, with three floors and mea-
suring 15,000 square feet. The customers are well taken
care of by young, fresh-faced college women who are
knowledgeable about what they are selling. There is also a
store in Montreal.

Specialty Items

For those of you who are interested in a few more items to jazz
up your sexual chemistry with your partner, check out these
products.

STS PEARL NECKLACES

These beautiful strands of pearls can be ordered through the
Sexuality Seminars e-mail address: rintonn@aol.com/ They are
available in a wide range of colors, incuding the standard white
and ivory pearl, and I recommend a 30″–36″ strand with a round
bead 8–10 mm. I also recommend a small clasp, or a strand with
none at all.

THE SOPHISTI-KIT™

I developed this all-inclusive kit in response to a request from seminar attendees. The result is a trademarked collection of products ranging from various lubricants to beautifully scented massage oils, games, vibrators, "rigatonis" and "calamaris," Pink Elephants, and pearl necklaces.

Ideal for wedding, anniversary, and bridal shower gifts, the kits can be custom designed in gift boxes. Included in any kit is a handout of ideas from the seminar. In a keepsake, white moiré–patterned hinged box, it is for discreet storage. You can order through e-mail at rintonn@aol.com/

BODY GEMS

For the girl who has everything, these exquisitely designed jewelry pieces become an aphrodisiac. Rather than merely decorate your body, they are designed for visual and tactile stimulation— just one more way to get him in the mood and raring to go. Body Gems are sensual, fresh, luxurious, fun, and decadent. They make good use of the intrigue and allure that is inherent in all gems. They can all be ordered via e-mail at rintonn@aol.com/

Passion Rubies: Historically rubies have been used to incite passion. These delicate gems can be spilled into a bubbling champagne flute, and as you and your lover watch them rise with the effervescence, the excitement will travel through you. Each gem contains one carat of genuine, faceted ruby, and they are packaged in award-winning style. $200.

BedPearls: These loose, lustrous, freshwater baroque pearls come wrapped in a love sonnet. Unwrap, shake, and throw the seven pearls onto your bed, slip them between the sheets, and then let them lure and excite you and your partner as you roll on a bed of pearls. $175.

SexPearls: This ten-foot strand of freshwater pearls can be wrapped, draped, or dragged over your body or his. Let them lie between your teeth, fall between your breasts, and glisten down the length of your leg. I guarantee it will drive him wild. $800.

FREE INFORMATION AND REFERRALS

Sexually Transmitted Diseases (STDs)

Centers for Disease Control
Public Health Service AIDS Hotline
800–342–AIDS, 24 hours a day, 7 days a week

STD National Hotline (Centers for Disease Control)
800–227–8922 8:00 a.m. to 11:00 p.m. (EST) weekdays

Hepatitis Hotline (Centers for Disease Control)
404–332–4555 extension 3
or The American Liver Foundation
1–800–223–0179

Herpes Resource Center
919–361–8488

Sexuality

American Association of Sex Educators, Counselors and
Therapists (AASECT)
319–897–8407

Can provide a list of AASECT certified therapists in your area.
Society for the Scientific Study of Sexuality (The 4Ss)
Same phone number as AASECT.

American Board of Sexology
1–800–533–3521

Can provide referrals to diplomates and clinical supervisors in
your area.

Any of the listed products in the book can be purchased through The Sexuality Seminars. All transactions are confidential and we do not sell our mailing list. Call 1–877–SexSeminars (1–877–739–7364) to:

- Purchase product (complete with instructions and suggestions for use)
- Book a seminar
- Get more information
- Be placed on the STS Newsletter mailing list
- Inquire about Lou Paget's seminar schedule

Purchases can be made by Visa, MasterCard, cash, or check. STS Los Angeles shows on bank statements. All product is discreetly packaged and shipped Priority Post unless otherwise requested. The Specialty Sophisti-Kits gift boxes can arrive in presentation style or closed—for a bigger surprise. They are delivered via UPS.

For more information, we can be reached at The STS Seminar Web site at:
wypwrs.com/adv/LPaget.html

For seminar inquiries, write to:
11601 Wilshire Blvd., Suite 500, Los Angeles, CA 90025
or
rintonn@aol.com